# Responding to Psychological Emergencies: A Field Guide

# Responding to Psychological Emergencies: A Field Guide

## Jeffrey A. Thomas, Psy.D.

Clinical Associate Professor
Arizona State University
City of Goodyear Fire Department
Goodyear, AZ

## S. Joseph Woodall, Ph.D.

Visiting Assistant Professor
University of North Carolina at Charlotte
Charlotte, NC

THOMSON
DELMAR LEARNING

Australia Canada Mexico Singapore Spain United Kingdom United States

**THOMSON**

**DELMAR LEARNING**

## Responding to Psychological Emergencies: A Field Guide
by Jeffrey A. Thomas, Psy.D., and S. Joseph Woodall, Ph.D.

**Vice President, Health Care Business Unit:**
William Brottmiller

**Director of Learning Solutions:**
Matthew Kane

**Acquisitions Editor:**
Maureen Rosener

**Product Manager:**
Elizabeth Howe

**Marketing Director:**
Jennifer McAvey

**Marketing Manager:**
Heather Sisley

**Marketing Coordinator:**
Christopher Manion

**Production Editor:**
Bridget Lulay

**Production Coordinator:**
Kenneth McGrath

For permission to use material from this text or product, contact us by
Tel (800) 730-2214
Fax (800) 730-2215
www.thomsonrights.com

**Library of Congress Cataloging-in-Publication Data**
Thomas, Jeffrey A.
    Responding to psychological emergencies : a field guide / Jeffrey A. Thomas, S. Joseph Woodall
        p. cm.
    Includes bibliographical references and index.
    ISBN 1-4018-7807-5 (alk. paper)
    1. Psychiatric emergencies—Handbooks, manuals, etc. I. Woodall, S. Joseph. II. Title.
    RC480.6.T47 2006
    616.89'025—dc22                      2005053712

### Notice to the Reader

Publisher does not warrant or guarantee any of the products described herein or perform any independent analysis in connection with any of the product information contained herein. Publisher does not assume, and expressly disclaims, any obligation to obtain and include information other than that provided to it by the manufacturer.

The reader is expressly warned to consider and adopt all safety precautions that might be indicated by the activities described herein and to avoid all potential hazards. By following the instructions contained herein, the reader willingly assumes all risks in connection with such instructions.

The publisher makes no representations or warranties of any kind, including but not limited to, the warranties of fitness for particular purpose or merchantability, nor are any such representations implied with respect to the material set forth herein, and the publisher takes no responsibility with respect to such material. The publisher shall not be liable for any special, consequential, or exemplary damages resulting, in whole or part, from the readers' use of, or reliance upon, this material.

# CONTENTS

## SECTION 2 Psychotropic Medications

## SECTION 3 Drugs of Abuse

## SECTION 4 Assessment

## SECTION 5 Reporting

## When Your Only Tool Is a Hammer, All Your Problems Look Like Nails

Many forces at work in society are perpetuating new challenges for emergency service workers and human services providers. These challenges are experienced out in the field in a variety of emergent and non-emergent settings. *Responding to Psychological Emergencies: A Field Guide* has been designed to add another tool to the professional's arsenal of tools as they are required to respond to an increasing number of these challenges.

The major goal of *Responding to Psychological Emergencies: A Field Guide* is to provide a user-friendly, cross-referenced, comprehensive, information resource for those delivering services. This reference source will assist those individuals first on the scene in making quick assessments and identifying intervention strategies that lie within their scope of practice.

This guide can be utilized as a rapid intervention tool that allows the user a variety of pathways to the desired information. Within thirty seconds of patient contact the user should be able to access vital information and intervention strategies that will enable the service provider to render a higher standard of care.

*Responding to Psychological Emergencies: A Field Guide* furnishes the professional with tools and information that enhance service delivery through successful assessment, intervention, and reporting of a host of issues. This guide contains a number of quality assessment tools, descriptions of psychological disorders, medications and medication interactions, drugs of abuse, and reporting strategies. It also is designed to provide foundational knowledge in the area of psychological emergencies.

It should be noted that the main focus of *Responding to Psychological Emergencies: A Field Guide* is the emergent and non-emergent field setting. Therefore, not every psychological disorder, social crisis, or drug of abuse is included. As a result of both research and experience, only those disorders that are most likely to be encountered in the field are included.

This guide is designed to meet the pressing needs of professionals and volunteers working in fire service, emergency medical services, law enforcement, detention and correctional facilities, hospital emergency rooms, crisis services, schools, private security, and disaster relief agencies. Virtually any service provider who encounters and serves others in the field setting should find this guide useful.

## Acknowledgments

The authors gratefully acknowledge the following individuals, agencies, and institutions for their assistance and support during the creation of this guide:

Jodi Woodall
Alexis Woodall
Lindsey Woodall
Drake Woodall
Andrew McCarthy
Captain Patrick Doyle, CEP
Sheldon Wagman, D.O.
Elizabeth Howe
Goodyear Fire Department
Peoria Fire Department
University of North Carolina at Charlotte—Division of Fire Safety Engineering Technology
Arizona State University—Fire Service Programs
Bruce Evans, NREMT-P, MPA
Thomson Delmar Learning

Special thanks are extended to the reviewers of this guide:
Harold C. Cohen, PhD, CHE, EMT-P, Baltimore County Fire Department
Bruce Evans, NREMT-P, MPA, Community College of Southern Nevada
Kristine Kern, LP, College of the Mainland
Christopher C. Miller, Hemet Fire Department
M. Jane Pollack, EMT-P, CEI, East Carolina University

This guide is designed for easy referencing. Subjects are divided into five major categories: 1) Psychological Emergencies, 2) Psychotropic Medications, 3) Drugs of Abuse, 4) Assessment, and 5) Reporting. Each section is color-coded and each subject is assigned an individual guide number to assist with referencing. Subjects located in the Introduction are assigned guide numbers 001–004. Subjects in Psychological Emergencies are assigned guide numbers 101–137. Psychotropic Medications are assigned guide numbers 201–255. Drugs of Abuse are assigned guide numbers 301–328. The different assessment tools located in the Assessment section are assigned guide numbers 401–410. Guides for Reporting have been assigned guide numbers 501–505. Each guide is intended to provide information that will aid in the rapid assessment of a patient's presenting problem. Each guide is cross-referenced with other guides to allow the professional to access additional information that may be of assistance.

Psychological Emergencies includes a combination of psychological disorders and social situations that are likely to create some type of medical, psychological, or social crisis for an individual. Psychotropic Medications includes a comprehensive list of medications that are prescribed in the treatment of psychological disorders. Drugs of Abuse contains a listing of various substances that are sometimes abused by members of society. The assessment tools located in Assessments are outlines designed to further the professional's ability to conduct a thorough evaluation of the patient. The Reporting section contains a number of tools that will serve to enhance a professional's ability to assess and report patient problems in a complete and systematic manner.

# WHAT IS A PSYCHOLOGICAL EMERGENCY?

## Definition

- An emotionally significant event or radical change of status in a person's life
- A crucial stage at which future events are determined

## Types of Psychological Emergencies

- Abuse
- Arrest or Detention
- Crime Victim
- Danger to Others
- Danger to Self
- Death
- Disasters
- Family Problems
- Fire
- Loss
- Medical Emergencies
- Psychological Disorders
- Substance Abuse
- Traumatic Events
- Victimization

## Factors That Affect Psychological Emergencies

- Age and development of the individual
- Whether the event is anticipated or unexpected
- Coping ability of the individual
- Current physical health status of the individual

- Current mental health status of the individual
- Duration of the event—long or short
- Educational level of the individual
- Individual perception of the event
- Pre-incident level of stress of the individual
- Previous life experiences of the individual
- Social support system of the individual
- Social, cultural, and ethnic background of the individual
- Spiritual or religious beliefs of the individual
- Violent or non-violent event
- Was the incident shared or was it individual
- Was there a threat to life
- What was lost during the event

INTRODUCTION

# Introduction

## GUIDE 001 — INTRODUCTION: ALPHABETICAL INDEX

### Introduction

## GUIDE 002 — PERSONAL PROTECTIVE EQUIPMENT (PPE)

### Description

- Body substances can pose a hazard to first responders and health care providers. Communicable diseases such as hepatitis B and C, HIV Disease, meningitis, pneumonia, mumps, tuberculosis, chicken pox, staphylococcus infection, and pertussis can be spread to individuals who do not properly protect themselves from exposure. The Centers for Disease Control and Prevention (CDC), the Occupational Safety and Health Administration (OSHA), and the National Fire Protection Association (NFPA) recommend that all first responders and health care providers use PPE.

### Personal Protective Equipment

- Disposable gloves
- Safety glasses or goggles
- High-efficiency particulate air (HEPA) mask
- Disposable sleeves
- Disposable gown
- Face shield

*Note: Wash hands or use an alcohol-based hand sanitizer after every patient contact*

## GUIDE 003 — APPROACHING PATIENTS

Several key factors must be a part of every patient contact.

### Unconditional Positive Regard

- Treat patients with dignity
- Be respectful

- Do not make judgments
- Understand that it is truly an emergency to them

## Introductions

- Always introduce yourself by giving them your name
- Tell them what your role and/or job title is
- Display your credentials if appropriate

## Addressing Patients

- Always ask patients their name
- Address adults as "Mr.," "Mrs.," "Miss," or "Ms."
- Use their first name if they give you permission

## Building Trust & Rapport

- Show empathy for the patient's situation
- Be supportive and reassuring
- Display a calm, compassionate, and caring attitude
- Be respectful of the patient's and the family's feelings

## Environment

- Always assess scene safety *Guide 402*
- Attend to the physical comfort of the patient
- Be aware of the temperature and the sun
- Provide water, blankets, and shade
- Be mindful of the patient's modesty needs
- Remove bystanders

## Confidentiality

- All patients expect the right to privacy with regard to psychological emergencies
- The patient's records must be kept confidential
- Always tell the patient what you are going to report and to whom
- Most emergency service, health care, and education professionals are mandated reporters of abuse *Guides 503, 504, 505*

## GUIDE 004 EMOTIONAL FIRST AID

### Definition

- A type of psychological intervention focused on helping a person to feel calm, safe, and well cared for during an acute, critical situation

## Methods

### Attending

Behaviors that let the patient know that you are paying attention to him or her:

- Maintain good eye contact
- Use the patient's name
- Refrain from charting or taking notes
- Give the patient your full attention

### Open-Ended Questions

Useful for gathering information regarding the emergency

- Ask questions that require more than a simple yes or no answer
- Example: "Tell me what has happened to you today."
- This encourages patients to talk freely

### Noncommittal Acknowledgments

Actions that let the patient know you are listening

- Nodding your head while the person is talking
- Vocalizations such as "ah," "uh-huh," and "hmmm"
- Responding with comments such as "yes," "I'm listening," and "okay"

### Door Openers

Comments that encourage the patient to share more

- "Tell me more"
- "Help me understand that"
- "Explain that to me"

### Content Paraphrase

Remarks that let the patient know that you understand what he or she has been saying

- Summarize what the patient has told you
- Use quotes if appropriate

### Silence

- This allows the patient time to collect his or her thoughts
- Do not feel as though you must fill up the silence
- If the silence is prolonged, try an open-ended question

### Self-Disclosure

Disclosing to the patient what is happening for you at that very moment

*Examples*
- "I'm confused"
- "I don't understand"
- "I'm concerned about you"
- "I want to help you"

*Note: It is inappropriate and unprofessional to share personal stories from your own life*

### Active Listening

Listening for and identifying the emotional tone of what a patient is saying

- Reflect the feeling back to the patient
- If you are incorrect, the patient will correct you

*Examples*
  - "You sound angry"
  - "You're frightened"
  - "I hear the sadness in your voice"

*Note: Never tell patients they should not feel the way they do*

### Providing Resources

- Any source of aid or support that can be provided to the patient
- Obtain or develop a resource list that is specific to your community

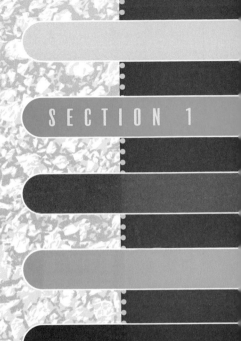

SECTION 1

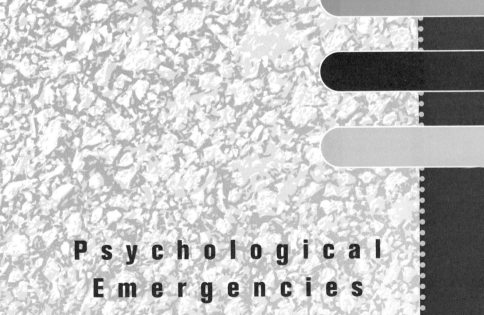

# Psychological Emergencies

# GUIDE 101   PSYCHOLOGICAL EMERGENCIES: ALPHABETICAL INDEX

1

1

## GUIDE 102 ACUTE STRESS DISORDER

### Description

- Symptoms develop within 1 month after exposure to an extremely traumatic stressor or event
- Symptoms interfere with daily functioning
- Symptoms are not the result of other psychological disorders

### Signs & Symptoms

- Subjective sense of numbing or detachment

- Decreased emotional response
- Depersonalization
- Difficulty concentrating
- Feelings of guilt
- Trauma is often re-experienced through thoughts, dreams, and/or flashbacks

## Assessment

- Assess scene safety *Guide 402*
- Use personal protective equipment (PPE) *Guide 002*
- Approach patient *Guide 003*
- Primary and secondary medical survey *Guide 403*

- Medications and compliance
- Brief mental status exam *Guide 404*
- Brief psychosocial history *Guide 405*
- Emotional first aid *Guide 004*

## Reporting

- Description of patient
- Chief complaint
- Medical findings
- Medications and compliance
- Mental status
- Psychosocial history

---

## GUIDE 103 — ATTENTION DEFICIT DISORDER (ADD)/ATTENTION DEFICIT HYPERACTIVITY DISORDER (ADHD)

### Description

- Chronic neurological condition
- Usually present since birth
- Hyperactivity may or may not be present
- Accompanying depression is also common
- Substance abuse may also be a problem

### Signs & Symptoms

*Attention*

- Easily distracted
- Has difficulty following instructions
- Disorganized
- Forgetful; loses things easily
- Inattentive to details

*Hyperactivity*

- Has difficulty remaining still
- Fidgets
- Talks excessively
- Abnormal sleep patterns

*Impulsivity*

- Impatient
- Often interrupts
- Acts without thinking first

## Medications

### Amphetamines (Adderall, Dexedrine) Guide 202
- Central nervous system (CNS) stimulant
- Generic available
- Addictive

### Antidepressants — Tricyclic Guide 203
- Antidepressants-Trycyclic
- Generic available
- Nonaddictive

### Atomoxetine (Strattera) Guide 208
- Selective norepinephrine reuptake inhibitor
- Generic not available
- Nonaddictive
- Appears to block a chemical neurotransmitter in the brain having to do with attention and activity

### Bupropion (Wellbutrin) Guide 213
- Antidepressant
- No generic available
- Nonaddictive

### Methylphenidate (Concerta, Metadate, Ritalin) Guide 234
- CNS stimulant
- Generic available
- Addictive

### Pemoline Guide 243
- CNS stimulant
- No generic available
- Addictive

## Assessment
- Assess scene safety Guide 402
- Use PPE Guide 002
- Approach patient Guide 003
- Primary and secondary medical survey Guide 403
- Medications and compliance
- Brief mental status exam Guide 404
- Brief psychosocial history Guide 405
- Emotional first aid Guide 004

## Reporting
- Patient description
- Chief complaint
- Medical findings
- Medications and compliance
- Known diagnoses
- Mental status
- Psychosocial history

## ( GUIDE 104 ) ALZHEIMER'S DISEASE

### Description
- Gradual decline of cognitive functions
- Multiple cognitive deficits
- Deficits cause significant impairment in functioning

- More common after age 65
- Prevalence increases sharply after age 75

## Signs & Symptoms

- Memory impairment
- Confabulation—the invention of facts to replace memory gaps
- Aphasia—language disturbances
- Apraxia—impaired motor functions
- Agnosia—failure to recognize or identify objects
- Disturbance in executive functions: planning, organizing, sequencing, abstracting

## Medications

*Antihistamines: Diphenhydramine Guide 205*

- Antihistamine
- Generic available
- Nonaddictive

*Cholinesterase Inhibitors (Aricept, Cognex, Exelon, Razadyne) Guide 218*

- Cholinesterase inhibitor

- No generic available
- Nonaddictive

## Assessment

- Assess scene safety *Guide 402*
- Use PPE *Guide 002*
- Approach patient *Guide 003*
- Primary and secondary medical survey *Guide 403*
- Medications and compliance
- Brief mental status exam *Guide 404*
- Brief psychosocial history *Guide 405*
- Emotional first aid *Guide 004*

## Reporting

- Description of patient
- Chief complaint
- Medical findings
- Medications and compliance
- Known diagnoses
- Mental status

# (GUIDE 105) AMNESIA

## Description

- Any partial or complete memory loss
- There are several types of amnesia

- May be caused by physiological factors such as stroke, trauma, other medical conditions

## Signs & Symptoms

- Disorientation may occur with profound amnesia
- Inability to recall events from the recent past
- Inability to recall events from the remote past
- Confabulation—the invention of facts to replace memory gaps
- Apathy
- Flat affect

## Assessment

- Assess scene safety *Guide 402*
- Use PPE *Guide 002*
- Approach patient *Guide 003*
- Primary and secondary medical surveys *Guide 403*
- Medications and compliance
- Brief mental status exam *Guide 404*
- Lethality assessment *Guide 407*
- Brief psychosocial history *Guide 405*
- Emotional first aid *Guide 004*

## Reporting

- Description of patient
- Chief complaint
- Medical findings
- Medications and compliance
- Known diagnoses
- Mental status
- Lethality
- Psychosocial history

# GUIDE 106 ANXIETY DISORDER

## Description

- Cover term for a number of disorders for which anxiety is the primary feature
- A vague, unpleasant emotional state with the qualities of apprehension, dread, distress, and uneasiness
- Causes significant impairment in ability to function

## Signs & Symptoms

- Chronic, unrealistic, and excessive anxiety and/or worry
- Restlessness
- Feeling "on edge"
- Fatigue
- Difficulty concentrating
- Irritability
- Sleep disturbances

## Medications

*Antidepressants—Tricyclic*
*Guide 203*

- Antidepressant
- Generic available
- Nonaddictive

### Aripiprazole (Abilify)
*Guide 207*
- Antipsychotic
- No generic available
- Nonaddictive
- Blocks certain impulses between nerve cells

### Barbiturates *Guide 209*
- Sedative: hypnotic, anticonvulsant
- Some generics available
- Addictive

### Benzodiazepines *Guide 210*
- Tranquilizer, anticonvulsant
- Generic available
- Addictive

### Beta-Blockers *Guide 211*
- Beta-adrenergic blocker
- Generic available
- Nonaddictive
- Diuretic: forces sodium and water excretion and relaxes muscle cells of small arteries

### Buspirone (BuSpar) *Guide 214*
- Antianxiety
- Generic available
- Addictive

### Ergotamine, Belladonna, & Phenobarbital *Guide 224*
- Analgesic, antispasmodic, vasoconstrictor
- Generic available
- Addictive

### Haloperidol (Haldol)
*Guide 226*
- Antipsychotic

- Generic available
- Nonaddictive

### Hydroxyzine *Guide 227*
- Tranquilizer, antihistamine
- Generic available
- Nonaddictive

### Loxapine (Loxitane) *Guide 230*
- Tranquilizer, antidepressant
- Generic available
- Nonaddictive

### Meprobamate *Guide 233*
- Tranquilizer, antianxiety
- Generic available
- Nonaddictive

### Molindone *Guide 237*
- Antipsychotic
- No generic available
- Nonaddictive
- Treats imbalance in nerve impulses from the brain

### Phenothiazines *Guide 245*
- Tranquilizer, antiemetic
- Some generics available
- Nonaddictive

### Selective Serotonin Reuptake Inhibitors (SSRIs) *Guide 249*
- Antidepressant, antiobsessional, antianxiety
- Some generics available
- Nonaddictive

### Thiothixene (Navane)
*Guide 251*
- Antipsychotic
- Generic available
- Nonaddictive

*Trazodone* Guide 253
- Antidepressant (nontri-cyclic) inhibits serotonin uptake in the brain
- Generic available
- Nonaddictive

*Venlafaxine (Effexor)* Guide 255
- Antidepressant—bicyclic
- No generic available
- Nonaddictive

## Assessment
- Assess scene safety *Guide 402*
- Use PPE *Guide 002*
- Approach patient *Guide 003*
- Primary and secondary medical survey *Guide 403*

- Medications
- Brief mental status exam *Guide 404*
- Brief psychosocial history *Guide 405*
- Emotional first aid *Guide 004*

## Reporting
- Description of patient
- Chief complaint
- Medical findings
- Medications and compliance
- Known diagnoses
- Mental status
- Psychosocial history

## (GUIDE 107) BIPOLAR DISORDER

### Description
- Also known as manic depression
- Cycling between phases of mania and depression
- Length of cycles varies
- Chronic and recurring
- Psychotic behavior often present in manic phase

### Signs & Symptoms
*Mania*
- Elevated mood
- Flight of ideas
- Hyperactivity
- Insomnia
- Delusions
- Grandiosity
- Poor judgment
- Aggression and/or hostility

*Depression*
- Depressed mood
- Loss of interest in pleasurable activities
- Feeling hopeless and/or helpless
- Appetite changes
- Sleep changes

## Medications

### Carbamazapine (Tegretol)
Guide 215
- Analgesic, anticonvulsant, antimanic
- Generic available
- Nonaddictive

### Divalproex (Depakote)
Guide 222
- Anticonvulsant
- No generic available
- Nonaddictive

### Lithium Guide 229
- Mood stabilizer
- Generic available
- Nonaddictive

### Olanzapine (Zyprexa)
Guide 241
- Antipsychotic
- No generic available
- Nonaddictive
- Blocks certain nerve impulses

### Valproic Acid (Depakene)
Guide 254
- Anticonvulsant
- Generic available
- Nonaddictive

## Assessment
- Assess scene safety Guide 402
- Use PPE Guide 002
- Approach patient Guide 003
- Primary and secondary medical survey Guide 403
- Medications and compliance
- Brief mental status exam Guide 404
- Lethality assessment Guide 407
- Brief psychosocial history Guide 405
- Emotional first aid Guide 004

## Reporting
- Description of patient
- Chief complaint
- Medical findings
- Medications and compliance
- Known diagnoses
- Mental status
- Lethality
- Psychosocial history

## GUIDE 108 CONDUCT DISORDER

### Description
- Individual repetitively and persistently violates the basic rights, privileges, and privacy of others
- Violates societal norms or rules
- Child onset: has one of the listed signs and symptoms prior to age 10

- Adolescent onset: manifests no signs or symptoms prior to age 10

## Signs & Symptoms

- Manifested by the presence of three or more of the following criteria in the past 12 months, with at least one criterion present in the past 6 months

### *Aggression Toward People and/or Animals*

- Bullies, threatens, or intimidates others
- Starts fights
- Used a harmful weapon
- Physically cruel to people
- Physically cruel to animals
- Stealing while confronting a victim: mugging, purse-snatching, extortion, armed robbery
- Forced sexual activity

### *Destruction of Property*

- Deliberately engaged in fire-setting with serious intent
- Deliberately destroyed property of others (not fire setting)

### *Deceitfulness or Theft*

- Broken into homes, cars, or businesses
- "Cons" others
- Stealing other items of importance: shoplifting but not breaking and entering

### *Serious Violations of Rules*

- Breaks curfew frequently
- Ran away from home at least twice while living under supervision, or once for a long period of time
- Skips school before age 13

## Medications

### *Aripiprazole (Abilify)*
*Guide 207*

- Antipsychotic
- No generic available
- Nonaddictive

### *Carbamazapine (Tegretol)*
*Guide 215*

- Analgesic, anticonvulsant, antimanic
- Generic available
- Nonaddictive

### *Clozapine (Clozaril) Guide 220*

- Antipsychotic
- Generic available
- Nonaddictive

### *Divalproex (Depakote)*
*Guide 222*

- Anticonvulsant
- No generic available
- Nonaddictive

### *Haloperidol (Haldol)*
*Guide 226*

- Antipsychotic
- Generic available
- Nonaddictive

### *Lithium Guide 229*

- Mood stabilizer

- Generic available
- Nonaddictive

*Molindone (Moban)* *Guide 237*

- Antipsychotic
- No generic available
- Nonaddictive

*Olanzapine (Zyprexa)* *Guide 241*

- Antipsychotic
- No generic available
- Nonaddictive

*Quetiapine (Seroquel)* *Guide 246*

- Antipsychotic
- No generic available
- Nonaddictive

*Risperidone (Risperdal)* *Guide 247*

- Antipsychotic
- No generic available
- Nonaddictive

*Valproic Acid (Depakene)* *Guide 254*

- Anticonvulsant
- Generic available
- Nonaddictive

## Assessment

- Assess scene safety *Guide 402*
- Use PPE *Guide 002*
- Approach patient *Guide 003*
- Primary and secondary medical survey *Guide 403*
- Medications and compliance
- Brief mental status exam *Guide 404*
- Brief psychosocial history *Guide 405*
- Emotional first aid *Guide 004*

## Reporting

- Description of patient
- Chief complaint
- Medical findings
- Medications and compliance
- Known diagnoses
- Mental status
- Psychosocial history

## GUIDE 109 CRIME VICTIM

### Description

- A person against whom a criminal offense has been committed
- Any family member of a person against whom a criminal offense has been committed

### Signs & Symptoms

*Physical*

- Bullet wounds
- Stab wounds
- Broken bones
- Strains or sprains

- Cuts, bruises, scrapes, and/or scratches
- Heart palpitations
- Tachycardia
- Hypertension
- Pressure in the chest
- Increased respirations

*Psychological*

- Anger, rage
- Contradictory behavior
- Denial
- Depression
- Fear, terror
- Frenzied activity
- Frustration
- Grief and sorrow
- Guilt and self-blame
- Immobility
- Regression
- Screaming, crying, hysterical outbursts
- Self-destructive or other violent acts
- Shock, disbelief, confusion

## Social Considerations

- Counseling/therapy costs
- Funeral costs
- Medical costs

- Missed work
- Property damage
- Stolen or missing property

## Assessment

- Assess scene safety *Guide 402*
- Use PPE *Guide 002*
- Approach victim *Guide 003*
- Primary and secondary medical survey *Guide 403*
- Medications and compliance
- Brief mental status exam *Guide 404*
- Lethality assessment *Guide 407*
- Emotional first aid *Guide 004*

## Reporting

- Description of patient
- Chief complaint
- Medical findings
- Medications and compliance
- Known diagnoses
- Mental status
- Lethality

## GUIDE 110  DEATH NOTIFICATION

## General Principles

- Whenever possible, make death notification in person
- Always make notification in pairs

- Must be made in a timely fashion
- Use plain language: always tell the person(s) that their loved one has "died"; avoid terms such as "passed away,"

"gone to rest," "we've lost them," and "gone to heaven"
- Be factual
- Be respectful and compassionate

## Preparation

### *Verify the Facts*

- Be able to describe the circumstances of the death
- Is there an investigation?
- Determine what information can and cannot be disclosed
- Ascertain the location of the body
- Understand the procedures used by the Medical Examiner
- Be aware of any cultural issues that may be a factor

### *Have Resources Available If Needed*

- List of local mortuaries
- Contact information for the Medical Examiner's Office
- Grief support groups
- Victim services
- Chaplain

## In-Person Notifications

- Introduce yourself and your partner
- Display credentials
- Make certain you have the right person(s)
- Ask them to sit down with you
- Make eye contact
- Relate the information in a calm, patient, and understanding manner
- Explain what happened in clear, concise, simple language
- Avoid jargon, acronyms, codes, or other professional terminology
- Answer questions tactfully and honestly
- Do not jeopardize an ongoing investigation
- Ask if there is anyone you can help them to contact
- Stay until someone else arrives

### *Private Residence*

- Ask if you can come in
- Determine if any one else is at home
- Ask if they would like them to be present

### *Hospital or Other Public Setting*

- Find a quiet, private area

## Long-Distance Notification

- Do not make notification by telephone if at all possible
- Request assistance from local authorities
- Provide them with as many facts as you can
- Leave them your name and contact information

## Telephone Notification

- Introduce yourself and tell them what agency you are with
- Make certain you have the right person(s)
- Ask if they have someone with them
- Ask if they would like them to be a part of the conversation
- Relate the information in a calm, patient, and understanding manner
- Explain what happened in clear, concise, simple language
- Avoid jargon, acronyms, codes, or other professional terminology
- Answer questions tactfully and honestly
- Do not jeopardize an ongoing investigation
- Ask if there is anyone you can help them to contact
- Stay on the phone until you are certain that they are calm
- Leave them your name and contact information

## Reactions

- Be prepared for a wide array of reactions
- Understand that men and women may react differently
- Appreciate that reactions vary greatly with respect to culture

## Anger

- Anger is a common reaction to a death notification
- Do not take it personally
- Tell them you understand their anger and are willing to listen
- Remain calm; this will help diffuse the situation
- Do not argue or tell them not to be angry
- Avoid being judgmental
- Remain with the person(s) until they are calm

## Assessment

- Assess scene safety
  *Guide 402*
- Approach person(s)
  *Guide 003*
- Vital signs
- Current health conditions and current medications
- Brief mental status exam
  *Guide 404*
- Lethality assessment
  *Guide 407*
- Emotional first aid
  *Guide 004*

## (GUIDE 111) DELIRIUM

### Description

- Disturbance of conscious-ness and cognition
- There are multiple causes
- Delirium can be substance-induced
- Delirium Tremens is caused by alcohol withdrawal

### Signs & Symptoms

- Disorientation
- Memory deficits
- Language disturbance
- Slurred speech
- Perceptual distortions

### Assessment

- Assess scene safety *Guide 402*

- Use PPE *Guide 002*
- Approach patient *Guide 003*
- Primary and secondary medical survey *Guide 403*
- Check for signs of intoxication
- Brief mental status exam *Guide 404*
- Emotional first aid *Guide 004*

### Reporting

- Description of patient
- Chief complaint
- Medical findings
- Mental status

## (GUIDE 112) DEMENTIA

### Description

- Gradual decline of cognitive functions
- Multiple cognitive deficits
- Deficits cause significant impairment in functioning
- More common after age 65
- Prevalence increases sharply after age 75

### Signs & Symptoms

- Reduced alertness
- Memory impairment

- Confabulation—the inven-tion of facts to replace memory gaps
- Aphasia—language disturbances
- Apraxia—impaired motor functions
- Agnosia—failure to recog-nize or identify objects
- Disturbance in executive functions—planning, organizing, sequencing, abstracting

## Medications

*Buspirone (BuSpar) Guide 214*
- Antianxiety
- Generic available
- Addictive

*Cholinesterase Inhibitors (Aricept, Cognex, Exelon, Razadyne) Guide 218*
- Cholinesterase inhibitors
- No generic available
- Nonaddictive

*Ergoloid Mesylates Guide 223*
- Ergot preparation
- Generic available
- Nonaddictive

*Haloperidol (Haldol) Guide 226*
- Antipsychotic
- Generic available
- Nonaddictive

## Assessment

- Assess scene safety *Guide 402*
- Use PPE *Guide 002*
- Approach patient *Guide 003*
- Primary and secondary medical survey *Guide 403*
- Medications and compliance
- Brief mental status exam *Guide 404*
- Brief psychosocial history *Guide 405*
- Emotional first aid *Guide 004*

## Reporting

- Description of patient
- Chief complaint
- Medical findings
- Medications and compliance
- Known diagnoses
- Mental status
- Psychosocial history

1

## GUIDE 113    DEPRESSION

### Description

- Mood state characterized by a sense of inadequacy, feelings of despondency, decreased activity, pessimism, and sadness
- In children and adolescents, the mood may be irritable rather then sad

### Signs & Symptoms

- Depressed or irritable mood
- Flat affect
- Diminished interest in pleasurable activities
- Significant weight change
- Insomnia or hypersomnia
- Psychomotor agitation

- Fatigue
- Feelings of worthlessness
- Feelings of guilt
- Feelings of hopelessness
- Difficulty concentrating
- Recurrent thoughts of death
- Suicidal ideation

## Medications

*Amphetamines—Elderly Patients* Guide 202
- CNS stimulant
- Generic available
- Addictive

*Antidepressants—Tricyclic* Guide 203
- Antidepressant
- Generic available
- Nonaddictive

*Bupropion (Wellbutrin)* Guide 213
- Antidepressant
- No generic available
- Nonaddictive

*Buspirone (BuSpar)* Guide 214
- Antianxiety
- Generic available
- Addictive

*Ergoloid Mesylates* Guide 223
- Ergot preparation
- Generic available
- Nonaddictive

*Loxapine* Guide 230
- Tranquilizer, antidepressant
- Generic available
- Nonaddictive

*Monoamine Oxidase (MAO) Inhibitors* Guide 231
- MAO inhibitor, antidepressant
- Generic available
- Nonaddictive

*Maprotiline (Ludiomil)* Guide 232
- Antidepressant
- Generic available
- Nonaddictive

*Methylphenidate (Concerta, Metadate, Ritalin)* Guide 234
- CNS stimulant
- Generic available
- Addictive

*Mirtazapine (Remeron)* Guide 235
- Antidepressant
- No generic available
- Nonaddictive

*Nefazodone (Serzone)* Guide 238
- Antidepressant
- No generic available
- Nonaddictive

*Selegiline* Guide 248
- Antidyskinetic
- Generic available
- Nonaddictive

*SSRIs* Guide 249
- Antidepressant, antiobsessional, antianxiety
- Some generics available
- Nonaddictive

*Trazodone* Guide 253
- Antidepressant
- Generic available
- Nonaddictive

*Venlafaxine (Effexor)*
Guide 255
- Antidepressant-bicyclic
- No generic available
- Nonaddictive

## Assessment

- Assess scene safety
  Guide 402
- Use PPE Guide 002
- Approach patient Guide 003
- Primary and secondary
  medical survey Guide 403
- Medications and
  compliance

- Brief mental status exam
  Guide 404
- Lethality assessment
  Guide 407
- Brief psychosocial history
  Guide 405
- Emotional first aid
  Guide 004

## Reporting

- Description of patient
- Chief complaint
- Medical findings
- Medications and
  compliance
- Known diagnoses
- Mental status
- Lethality
- Psychosocial history

1

---

## GUIDE 114   DISSOCIATIVE IDENTITY DISORDER

### Description

- Also known as multiple
  personality disorder
- Presence of two or more
  distinct identities or personality states
- Relatively rare disorder

### Signs & Symptoms

- Two or more distinct identities or personality states,
  each with its own enduring
  pattern of perceiving, relat-
  ing to, and thinking about
  the environment

- At least two of these identities or personality states
  recurrently take control of
  the patient's behavior
- Inability to recall personal
  information that is too
  extensive to be explained by
  ordinary forgetfulness

### Medications

*Antidepressants — Tricyclic*
Guide 203
- Antidepressant
- Generic available
- Nonaddictive

**Benzodiazepines** *Guide 210*
- Tranquilizer, anticonvulsant
- Generic available
- Addictive

**Buspirone (BuSpar)** *Guide 214*
- Antianxiety
- Generic available
- Addictive

**Loxapine (Loxitane)** *Guide 230*
- Tranquilizer, antidepressant
- Generic available
- Nonaddictive

**Monoamine Oxidase (MAO) Inhibitors** *Guide 231*
- MAO inhibitor, antidepressant
- Generic available
- Nonaddictive

**Maprotiline (Ludiomil)** *Guide 232*
- Antidepressant
- Generic available
- Nonaddictive

**Meprobamate** *Guide 233*
- Tranquilizer, antianxiety
- Generic available
- Nonaddictive

**Mirtazapine (Remeron)** *Guide 235*
- Antidepressant
- No generic available
- Nonaddictive

**Nefazodone (Serzone)** *Guide 238*
- Antidepressant
- No generic available
- Nonaddictive

**SSRIs** *Guide 249*
- Antidepressant, antiobsessional, antianxiety
- Some generics available
- Nonaddictive

**Trazodone** *Guide 253*
- Antidepressant
- Generic available
- Nonaddictive

**Venlafaxine (Effexor)** *Guide 255*
- Antidepressant-bicyclic
- No generic available
- Nonaddictive

## Assessment

- Assess scene safety *Guide 402*
- Use PPE *Guide 002*
- Approach patient *Guide 003*
- Primary and secondary medical survey *Guide 403*
- Medications and compliance
- Brief mental status exam *Guide 404*
- Lethality assessment *Guide 407*
- Brief psychosocial history *Guide 405*
- Emotional first aid *Guide 004*

## Reporting

- Description of patient
- Chief complaint
- Medical findings

- Medications and compliance
- Known diagnoses
- Mental status
- Lethality
- Psychosocial history

## (GUIDE 115) DOMESTIC VIOLENCE

### Description

- The use of physical violence, threats, emotional abuse, harassment, or stalking by spouses, intimate partners, or family members to control the behavior of their family members or partners

### Types of Domestic Violence

- Animal abuse
- Beating
- Biting
- Burning
- Harassment
- Hitting
- Humiliation
- Ignoring
- Insults
- Intimidation
- Isolation from family and friends
- Isolation from preferred activities
- Kicking
- Physical punishment
- Physical restraints
- Pinching
- Property destruction
- Pushing
- Shaking

- Shoving
- Stalking
- Striking—with or without an object
- The "silent treatment"
- Threats
- Verbal assaults
- Withholding medical treatment
- Unneeded or unwanted medical treatment

### Signs & Symptoms

*Physical*

- An individual reports being physically abused
- Black eyes
- Bone fractures
- Broken eyeglasses
- Bruises
- Cuts
- Dislocations
- Gastrointestinal disorders
- Internal injuries
- Headaches
- Lacerations
- Malnutrition
- Open wounds
- Punctures
- Rope marks
- Skull fractures
- Sleep disturbances

- Sprains
- Untreated injuries at various stages of healing
- Welts

*Psychological*

- Anger, rage
- Anxiety
- Contradictory behavior
- Denial
- Depression
- Fear, terror
- Frenzied activity
- Frustration
- Guilt and self-blame
- Immobility
- Post-traumatic stress
- Regression
- Running away
- Screaming, crying, hysterical outbursts
- Self-destructive or other violent acts
- Social withdrawal
- Suicide attempts

## Assessment

- Assess scene safety
  *Guide 402*

- Use PPE *Guide 002*
- Approach patient *Guide 003*
- Primary and secondary medical survey *Guide 403*
- Medications and compliance
- Brief mental status exam *Guide 404*
- Lethality assessment *Guide 407*
- Domestic violence screening *Guide 410*
- Brief psychosocial history *Guide 405*
- Emotional first aid *Guide 004*

## Reporting

- Description of patient
- Chief complaint
- Medical findings
- Medications and compliance
- Known diagnoses
- Mental status
- Lethality
- Domestic violence
- Psychosocial history

**GUIDE 116** EATING DISORDERS

## Description

- Severe disturbance in eating behavior

## Signs & Symptoms

*Anorexia nervosa*

- Refusal to maintain body weight at or above minimally normal weight

- Intense fear of gaining weight
- Disturbance in the way one's body weight or shape is perceived

### Females
- Amenorrhea—absence of three consecutive menstrual cycles without pregnancy

### Restricting Type
- Restricting food intake; may engage in purging behavior (i.c., vomiting and/or the misuse of laxatives, diuretics, or enemas)

### Binge Eating/Purging Type
- Regularly engages in binge eating and purging behavior (i.e., vomiting and/or the misuse of laxatives, diuretics, or enemas)

### Bulimia Nervosa
- Recurrent episodes of binge eating characterized by (1) eating an abnormally large amount of food during a discrete period of time and (2) a lack of control over eating during the episode
- Recurrent and inappropriate compensatory behavior following the binge (i.e., vomiting and/or the misuse of laxatives, diuretics, or enemas; fasting; and/or excessive exercise)
- Signs of depression Guide 113

### Purging Type
- Regularly engages in binge eating and purging behavior (i.e., vomiting and/or the misuse of laxatives, diuretics, or enemas)

### Nonpurging Type
- Recurrently and inappropriately engages in compensatory behavior following the binge (i.e., fasting and/or excessive exercise), but has not regularly engaged in purging behavior(i.e., vomiting and/or the misuse of laxatives, diuretics, or enemas)

## Medications

### Antidepressants—Tricyclic
Guide 203
- Antidepressant
- Generic available
- Nonaddictive

### SSRIs Guide 249
- Antidepressant, antiobsessional, antianxiety
- Some generics available
- Nonaddictive

## Assessment
- Assess scene safety Guide 402
- Use PPE Guide 002
- Approach patient Guide 003
- Primary and secondary medical survey Guide 403

- Medications and compliance
- Brief mental status exam
  *Guide 404*
- Lethality assessment
  *Guide 407*
- Brief psychosocial history
  *Guide 405*
- Emotional first aid
  *Guide 004*

## Reporting

- Description of patient
- Chief complaint
- Medical findings
- Medications and compliance
- Known diagnoses
- Mental status
- Lethality
- Psychosocial history

## ( GUIDE 117 ) GRIEF

### Description

- An intense emotional state associated with the loss of someone or something of significance
- Every person will grieve in a unique and individual way
- Every person will grieve at a different pace
- Each individual's grief will be affected by his or her own life history
- Grief typically lasts 2-3 years or more

### *Types of Losses*

- Loved one—spouse, significant other, child, parent, sibling, other relative, friend, pet, and so on
- Significant relationships—marriage or domestic partnership, friendship, employment, and so on
- Property—home, automobile, money, personal items, and so on
- Community—neighborhood, school, place of worship, clubs, associations, colleagues, and so on
- Line of Duty Losses—Emergency Medical Service, Fire Service, Law Enforcement, Military, Search and Rescue

### Signs & Symptoms

#### *Physical*

- Heart palpitations
- Hypertension
- Pressure in the chest
- Confusion
- Changes in appetite
- Digestive problems
- Dizziness
- Dry mouth
- Fatigue

- Headache
- Muscular pain
- Sleep disturbances

### Psychological

- Anger
- Anxiety
- Despair
- Difficulty concentrating
- Feeling a loss of control
- Feeling powerless and/or helpless
- Feelings of abandonment
- Feelings of loss
- Guilt
- Intense dreams
- Memory problems
- Sadness

## Factors Affecting Grief

### Physical

- Age
- Current health status
- Sleep patterns
- Diet and nutrition
- Digestion and elimination
- Exercise
- Sexual activity
- Caffeine intake
- Alcohol use
- Tobacco use
- Drug use

### Psychological

- Current mental health status
- Anticipated loss
- Coping behaviors

- Current level of concurrent stress
- Length of illness prior to death
- Level of education
- Loss was preventable
- Maturity level
- Personality
- Previous experience with loss
- Quality of the relationship
- Secondary losses
- Significance of loss
- Social, cultural, and ethnic background
- Spiritual and/or religious beliefs
- Sudden or unexpected loss
- Unfinished business

### Social

- Social support system
- Socioeconomic status
- Ethnic background
- Spiritual and/or religious beliefs
- Level of education
- Funeral practices/rituals

## Assessment

- Assess scene safety *Guide 402*
- Use PPE *Guide 002*
- Approach person(s) *Guide 003*
- Primary and secondary medical survey *Guide 403*
- Medications and compliance

- Brief mental status exam
  *Guide 404*
- Lethality assessment
  *Guide 407*

- Brief psychosocial history
  *Guide 405*
- Emotional first aid
  *Guide 004*

## (GUIDE 118) HOMELESSNESS

### Description

- A person who lacks a fixed, regular, and adequate night-time residence and has a primary night-time residence that is: (1) a supervised public or private shelter that is designed to provide temporary accommodations, (2) an institution that provides temporary residence for persons intended to be institutionalized, or (3) a public or private place not designed for or ordinarily used as a sleeping place for human beings

*The term "homelessness" does not apply to individuals who are incarcerated or imprisoned.*

### Reasons for Homelessness

- Poverty
- Unemployment
- Lack of public assistance
- Lack of affordable housing
- Lack of affordable health care
- Domestic violence
- Mental illness
- Substance abuse

### Assessment

- Assess scene safety
  *Guide 402*
- Use PPE *Guide 002*
- Approach patient *Guide 003*
- Primary and secondary medical survey *Guide 403*
- Medications and compliance
- Brief mental status exam
  *Guide 404*
- Lethality assessment
  *Guide 407*
- Brief psychosocial history
  *Guide 405*
- Emotional first aid
  *Guide 004*
- Provide resources for emergency shelter

### Reporting

- Description of patient
- Chief complaint
- Medical findings
- Medications and compliance
- Known diagnoses
- Mental status
- Lethality
- Brief psychosocial history

## Description

- The killing of a human being by one or more other human beings
- Surviving family and/or friends

## Signs & Symptoms

*Physical*

- Heart palpitations
- Tachycardia
- Hypertension
- Pressure in the chest
- Increased respiration

*Psychological*

- Anger, rage
- Contradictory behavior
- Denial
- Depression
- Fear, terror
- Frenzied activity
- Frustration
- Grief and sorrow
- Guilt and self-blame
- Immobility
- Regression
- Screaming, crying, hysterical outbursts
- Self-destructive or other violent acts
- Shock, disbelief, confusion

*Social*

- Counseling/therapy costs
- Funeral costs
- Medical costs
- Missed work

## Survivor Care

- Answer questions tactfully and honestly
- Ask if there is anyone you can help them to contact
- Avoid jargon, acronyms, codes, or other professional terminology
- Avoid judgments
- Be prepared to handle the grief reaction *Guide 117*
- Do not jeopardize an ongoing investigation
- Explain the role of the Medical Examiner
- Explain what happened in clear, concise, simple language
- Never leave the survivor(s) alone
- Relate the information in a calm, patient, and understanding manner
- Respect social, cultural, and ethnic traditions
- Screen survivors from the media
- Stay until someone else arrives
- Treat the body with respect
- Try to put yourself in the survivor's place—have a caring attitude

## Assessment

- Assess scene safety *Guide 402*

- Use PPE *Guide 002*
- Approach survivor(s)
  *Guide 003*
- Primary and secondary
  medical survey *Guide 403*
- Medications and compli-
  ance
- Brief mental status exam
  *Guide 404*
- Lethality assessment
  *Guide 407*
- Emotional first aid
  *Guide 004*

### Reporting

- Description of patient
- Chief complaint
- Medical findings
- Medications and
  compliance
- Known diagnoses
- Mental status
- Lethality

## GUIDE 120  HYPOCHONDRIASIS

### Description

- Preoccupation with the fear
  of the idea that one has a
  serious disease
- Based on the patient's mis-
  interpretation of bodily
  symptoms
- Condition persists despite
  appropriate medical evaluation and reassurance

### Signs & Symptoms

- Not of delusional intensity
- Not restricted to a circumscribed concern about
  appearance
- Causes clinically significant
  distress or impairment in
  social, occupational, or
  other important areas of
  functioning
- Duration of at least 6
  months

- Not better accounted for by
  another mental disorder

### Assessment

- Assess scene safety
  *Guide 402*
- Use PPE *Guide 002*
- Approach patient *Guide 003*
- Primary and secondary
  medical survey *Guide 403*
- Medications and
  compliance
- Brief mental status exam
  *Guide 404*
- Brief psychosocial history
  *Guide 405*
- Emotional first aid
  *Guide 004*

### Reporting

- Description of patient
- Chief complaint

- Medical findings
- Medications and compliance

- Known diagnoses
- Mental status
- Psychosocial history

## (GUIDE 121) NARCOLEPSY

### Description

- Repeated uncontrollable attacks of sleep
- Usually occurs daily

### Signs & Symptoms

- Daily attacks of uncontrollable sleep
- Cataplexy—brief episodes of bilateral loss of muscle tone
- Transient visual hallucinations at the beginning or end of sleep
- Sleep paralysis at the beginning or end of sleep

### Medications

*Amphetamines (Adderall, Dexedrine) Guide 202*

- CNS stimulant
- Generic available
- Addictive

*Antidepressants—Tricyclic Guide 203*

- Generic available
- Nonaddictive

*Methylphenidate (Concerta, Metadate, Ritalin) Guide 234*

- CNS stimulant
- Generic available
- Addictive

*Modafinil (Provigil) Guide 236*

- Antinarcoleptic CNS stimulant
- No generic available
- Addictive

### Assessment

- Assess scene safety *Guide 402*
- Use PPE *Guide 002*
- Approach patient *Guide 003*
- Primary and secondary medical survey *Guide 403*
- Medications and compliance
- Brief mental status exam *Guide 404*
- Brief psychosocial history *Guide 405*
- Emotional first aid *Guide 004*

### Reporting

- Description of patient
- Chief complaint
- Medical findings
- Medications and compliance
- Known diagnoses
- Mental status
- Psychosocial history

## Description

- Subclass of anxiety disorder
- Two essential characteristics: recurrent and persistent thoughts, ideas, and feelings; and repetitive, ritualized behaviors
- Attempts to resist a compulsion produce mounting tension and anxiety

## Signs & Symptoms

### Obsessions

- Intrusive and inappropriate thoughts, impulses, or images that cause marked anxiety or distress
- Not simply worries about real-life problems
- Has made attempts to neutralize with other thoughts or actions
- Patient recognizes that the thoughts, images, or impulses are products of his or her own mind

### Compulsions

- Repetitive behaviors—hand washing, ordering, checking, and so on—that patient is driven to perform according to strict rules/procedures
- Mental acts—praying, counting, repeating words silently, and so on—that the patient is driven to perform according to strict rules/procedures
- At some point, the patient has recognized that these behaviors/acts are excessive or unreasonable
- Takes more than 1 hour a day from normal activities
- Interferes significantly with normal routine, occupational or academic functioning, and/or social activities or relationships
- Not due to the impacts of a substance or general medical condition

## Medications

### Antidepressants—Tricyclic Guide 203

- Antidepressant
- Generic available
- Nonaddictive

### Benzodiazepines Guide 210

- Tranquilizer, anticonvulsant
- Generic available
- Addictive

### Buspirone (BuSpar) Guide 214

- Antianxiety
- Generic available
- Addictive

### Lithium Guide 229

- Mood stabilizer
- Generic available
- Nonaddictive

**SSRIs** *Guide 249*

- Antidepressant, antiobses-
  sional, antianxiety
- Some generics available
- Nonaddictive

### Assessment

- Assess scene safety
  *Guide 402*
- Use PPE *Guide 002*
- Approach patient *Guide 003*
- Primary and secondary
  medical survey *Guide 403*
- Medications and
  compliance
- Brief mental status exam
  *Guide 404*

- Brief psychosocial history
  *Guide 405*
- Emotional first aid
  *Guide 004*

### Reporting

- Description of patient
- Chief complaint
- Medical findings
- Medications and
  compliance
- Known diagnoses
- Mental status
- Psychosocial history

---

**GUIDE 123** OPPOSITIONAL DEFIANT DISORDER (ODD)

### Description

- Disorder of childhood and
  adolescence
- Pattern of negativistic, hostile, deviant behavior
- At least 6 months in
  duration

### Signs & Symptoms

- Frequent loss of temper
- Argues with authority
  figures
- Defies or refuses to comply
  with adult directives/rules
- Intentionally annoying
- Blames others for mistakes
- Easily annoyed/irritated
- Frequently angry and
  resentful

- Frequently spiteful or
  vindictive
- Actions impair social, academic, or occupational
  function

### Assessment

- Assess scene safety
  *Guide 402*
- Use PPE *Guide 002*
- Approach patient *Guide 003*
- Primary and secondary
  medical survey *Guide 403*
- Medications and
  compliance
- Brief mental status exam
  *Guide 404*
- Brief psychosocial history
  *Guide 405*

## Reporting
- Description of patient
- Chief complaint
- Medical findings
- Medications and compliance
- Known diagnoses
- Mental status
- Psychosocial history

## GUIDE 124 — PANIC DISORDER/PANIC ATTACK

### Description
- Discrete period of intense fear or discomfort, in which four or more of the signs and symptoms developed abruptly and reached a peak within 10 minutes

### Signs & Symptoms
- Palpitations, pounding heart, or tachycardia
- Perspiration
- Trembling or shaking
- Shortness of breath
- Smothering sensation
- Chest pain—discomfort
- Nausea—abdominal distress
- Dizziness, unsteadiness, lightheadedness, or faintness
- Derealization—feelings of unreality
- Depersonalization-feelings of being detached from oneself
- Fear of losing control or going crazy
- Fear of dying
- Paresthesias—numbness or tingling sensations
- Chills or hot flashes

### Medications
*Antidepressants—Tricyclic* Guide 203
- Antidepressant
- Generic available
- Nonaddictive

*Benzodiazepines* Guide 210
- Tranquilizer, anticonvulsant
- Generic available
- Addictive

*Monoamine Oxidase (MAO) Inhibitors* Guide 231
- MAO inhibitor, antidepressant
- Generic available
- Nonaddictive

### Assessment
- Assess scene safety Guide 402
- Use PPE Guide 002
- Approach patient Guide 003
- Primary and secondary medical survey Guide 403
- Medications and compliance
- Brief mental status exam Guide 404

- Brief psychosocial history
  *Guide 405*
- Emotional first aid
  *Guide 004*

### Reporting
- Description of patient
- Chief complaint

- Medical findings
- Medications and
  compliance
- Known diagnoses
- Mental status
- Psychosocial history

## (GUIDE 125) PARANOIA

### Description
- Pervasive distrust and suspiciousness of others

### Signs & Symptoms
- Unfounded suspicion of others
- Unjustified questioning of loyalty and trust of family and/or friends
- Reluctant to confide for fear of retribution
- Perceives hidden or threatening meaning in general communications
- Bears grudges
- Unforgiving

### *Severe*

Includes all of the above, plus the following:

- Preoccupation with one or more delusions
- Auditory hallucinations
- Does not present with disorganized speech or behavior, flat or inappropriate affect

### Medications

*Aripiprazole (Abilify)*
*Guide 207*
- Antipsychotic
- No generic available
- Nonaddictive

*Carbamazepine (Tegretol)*
*Guide 215*
- Analgesic, anticonvulsant, antimanic
- Generic available
- Nonaddictive

*Clozapine (Clozaril)* *Guide 220*
- Antipsychotic
- Generic available
- Nonaddictive

*Haloperidol (Haldol)*
*Guide 226*
- Antipsychotic
- Generic available
- Nonaddictive

*Molindone (Moban)* *Guide 237*
- Antipsychotic
- No generic available
- Nonaddictive

### Olanzapine (Zyprexa)
*Guide 241*
- Antipsychotic
- No generic available
- Nonaddictive

### Phenothiazines *Guide 245*
- Tranquilizer, antiemetic
- Generic available
- Nonaddictive

### Quetiapine (Seroquel)
*Guide 246*
- Antipsychotic
- No generic available
- Nonaddictive

### Risperidone (Risperdal)
*Guide 247*
- Antipsychotic
- No generic available
- Nonaddictive

### Thiothixene *Guide 251*
- Antipsychotic
- Generic available
- Nonaddictive
- Correction of nerve impulses

### Assessment
- Assess scene safety *Guide 402*
- Use PPE *Guide 002*
- Approach patient *Guide 003*
- Primary and secondary medical survey *Guide 403*
- Medications and compliance
- Brief mental status exam *Guide 404*
- Brief psychosocial history *Guide 405*
- Emotional first aid *Guide 004*

### Reporting
- Description of patient
- Chief complaint
- Medical findings
- Medications and compliance
- Known diagnoses
- Mental status
- Psychosocial history

---

## GUIDE 126   PARKINSON'S DISEASE

### Description
- Slowly progressive neuro-logical condition
- Dementia occurs in 20%-60% of patients
- Multiple cognitive deficits
- Deficits cause significant impairment in functioning

### Signs & Symptoms
- Tremor
- Muscular rigidity
- Bradykinesia—slowed movements
- Postural instability
- Cognitive slowing

- Disturbance in executive functions—planning, organizing, sequencing, abstracting
- Memory impairment
- Apraxia—impaired motor functions

## Medications

*Antidyskinetics* Guide 204
- Antidyskinetic, antiparkinsonism, dopamine agonists
- Generic available
- Nonaddictive

*Antihistamines* Guide 205
- Antihistamine
- Generic available
- Nonaddictive

*Antivirals for Influenza* Guide 206
- Antiviral, antiparkinsonism
- Generic available
- Nonaddictive

*Bromocriptine* Guide 212
- Antiparkinsonism
- Generic available
- Nonaddictive

*Carbidopa and Levodopa (Sinemet)* Guide 216
- Antiparkinsonism
- Generic available
- Nonaddictive

*Levodopa* Guide 228
- Antiparkinsonism
- Generic available
- Nonaddictive

*Niacin (Vitamin B-3)* Guide 240
- Vitamin supplement, vasodilator, antihyperlipidemic
- Generic available
- Nonaddictive

*Orphenadrine* Guide 242
- Muscle relaxant, anticholinergic, antihistamine, antiparkinsonism
- Generic available
- Possibly addictive

*Pergolide (Permax)* Guide 244
- Antidyskinetic
- No generic available
- Nonaddictive

*Selegiline* Guide 248
- Antidyskinetic
- Generic available
- Nonaddictive

*Tolcapone (Tasmar)* Guide 252
- Antidyskinetic, antiparkinsonism
- No generic available
- Nonaddictive

## Assessment

- Assess scene safety *Guide 402*
- Use PPE *Guide 002*
- Approach patient *Guide 003*
- Primary and secondary medical survey *Guide 403*
- Medications and compliance
- Brief mental status exam *Guide 404*

- Brief psychosocial history
  *Guide 405*
- Emotional first aid
  *Guide 004*

## Reporting

- Description of patient
- Chief complaint

- Medical findings
- Medications and compliance
- Known diagnoses
- Mental status
- Psychosocial history

## (GUIDE 127) PERSONALITY DISORDERS

### Description

- Class of behavioral disorders manifested as pathological developments in overall personality
- An enduring pattern of inner experience and behavior that greatly deviates from the expectations of the patient's culture
- Pervasive and inflexible
- Marked by little anxiety or distress

### Signs & Symptoms

- Onset in adolescence or early adulthood
- Pattern is stable over time
- Pattern is inflexible and pervasive across a broad range of personal and social situations
- Significant clinical distress and impairment in social, occupational, or other important areas of functioning

- Deviation in cognition of self, other people, and events
- Deviation in the range, intensity, lability, and appropriateness of emotional response
- Deviation in appropriate interpersonal functioning
- Poor impulse control
- Not a consequence of another mental disorder
- Not a consequence of drug abuse, medication, or a general condition such as head trauma

### Medications

*Benzodiazepines* Guide 210
- Tranquilizer, anticonvulsant
- Generic available
- Addictive

*Lithium* Guide 229
- Mood stabilizer
- Generic available
- Nonaddictive

*Monoamine Oxidase (MAO) Inhibitors* Guide 231

- MAO inhibitor, antidepressant
- Generic available
- Nonaddictive

*SSRIs* Guide 249

- Antidepressant, antiobsessional, antianxiety
- Some generics available
- Nonaddictive

*Valproic Acid* Guide 254

- Anticonvulsant
- Generic available
- Nonaddictive

## Assessment

- Assess scene safety Guide 402
- Use PPE Guide 002

- Approach patient Guide 003
- Primary and secondary medical survey Guide 403
- Medications and compliance
- Brief mental status exam Guide 404
- Brief psychosocial history Guide 405
- Emotional first aid Guide 004

## Reporting

- Description of patient
- Chief complaint
- Medical findings
- Medications and compliance
- Known diagnoses
- Mental status
- Psychosocial history

---

## GUIDE 128 — PERSON(S) DISPLACED FROM HOME BY CRIME, FIRE, OR OTHER DISASTER

### Description

- Person(s) who are unable to continue living in their residence because of a crime, fire, natural or man-made disaster, or emergency evacuation

### Signs & Symptoms

*Physical*

- Heart palpitations
- Tachycardia
- Hypertension
- Pressure in the chest
- Increased respiration

*Psychological*

- Anger, rage
- Contradictory behavior
- Denial
- Depression
- Fear, terror
- Frenzied activity
- Frustration
- Grief and sorrow
- Guilt and self-blame

- Immobility
- Regression
- Screaming, crying, hysterical outbursts
- Self-destructive or other violent acts
- Shock, disbelief, confusion

*Social*
- Housing costs
- Clothing costs
- Food costs
- Personal care item costs
- Missed work

## Survivor Care
- Answer questions tactfully and honestly
- Ask if there is anyone you can help them to contact
- Avoid jargon, acronyms, codes, or other professional terminology
- Avoid judgments
- Be prepared to handle the grief reaction *Guide 117*
- Explain what happened in clear, concise, simple language
- Never leave the survivor(s) alone
- Provide access to a telephone
- Provide resources for temporary shelter
- Relate the information in a calm, patient, and understanding manner

- Respect social, cultural, and ethnic traditions
- Screen survivors from the media
- Stay until someone else arrives
- Try to put yourself in the survivor's place—have a caring attitude

## Assessment
- Assess scene safety *Guide 402*
- Use PPE *Guide 002*
- Approach person(s) *Guide 003*
- Primary and secondary medical survey *Guide 403*
- Medications and compliance
- Brief mental status exam *Guide 404*
- Lethality assessment *Guide 407*
- Emotional first aid *Guide 004*

## Reporting
- Description of patient
- Chief complaint
- Medical findings
- Medications and compliance
- Known diagnoses
- Mental status
- Lethality

## Description

- Persistent and intense fear of an object or situation, with a compelling need to flee or avoid the source
- Fear is irrational and not based on sound judgment
- More common in women than men

## Signs & Symptoms

- Sudden onset of inner preoccupation with intense fear
- Shaking
- Tachycardia
- Hyperventilation
- Difficulty communicating
- Incoherent speech

### Agoraphobia

- Fear of leaving a secure base—typically the patient's home
- Most commonly reported phobia
- Deep fear of being caught alone in some public place
- Not better accounted for by another mental disorder, drug abuse, or medical condition
- Types include fear of being outside—being alone outside the home; being in a crowd; standing in line; being on a bridge; traveling in a bus, train, or automobile

### Specific Phobia

- Marked and persistent fear of clearly discernible, circumscribed objects or situations
- Exposure to the phobic stimulus invariably provokes an anxiety response
- Types include fear of animals, heights, storms, water, blood, injections, airplanes, elevators, and enclosed spaces

### Social Phobia

- Marked or persistent fear of one or more social or performance situations in which the patient is exposed to unfamiliar people or scrutiny by others
- Exposure to the phobic stimulus provokes an anxiety response
- Person recognizes that the fear is excessive or unreasonable
- Reaction interferes significantly with normal routine, occupational or academic functioning, social activities, or relationships
- Most common types are fear of public speaking, fear of crowds, fear of eating in public

## Medications

### Antidepressants — Tricyclic
*Guide 203*
- Antidepressant
- Generic available
- Nonaddictive

### Benzodiazepines *Guide 210*
- Tranquilizer, anticonvulsant
- Generic available
- Addictive

### Buspirone (BuSpar) *Guide 214*
- Antianxiety
- Generic available
- Addictive

### Loxapine *Guide 230*
- Tranquilizer, antidepressant
- Generic available
- Nonaddictive

### SSRIs *Guide 249*
- Antidepressant, antiobsessional, antianxiety
- Some generics available
- Nonaddictive

### Venlafaxine (Effexor)
*Guide 255*
- Antidepressant—bicyclic
- No generic available
- Nonaddictive

## Assessment
- Assess scene safety *Guide 402*
- Use PPE *Guide 002*
- Approach patient *Guide 003*
- Primary and secondary medical survey *Guide 403*
- Medications and compliance
- Brief mental status exam *Guide 404*
- Brief psychosocial history *Guide 405*
- Emotional first aid *Guide 004*

## Reporting
- Description of patient
- Chief complaint
- Medical findings
- Medications and compliance
- Known diagnoses
- Mental status
- Psychosocial history

## GUIDE 130 — POST-TRAUMATIC STRESS DISORDER (PTSD)

### Description
- Type of anxiety disorder
- Emerges after a psychologically distressing, traumatic event such as disaster, accident, war, or rape

### Signs & Symptoms
- Re-experiencing the trauma in dreams, recurrent thoughts and images
- Psychological numbness
- Detachment from world

- Hypervigilance
- Exaggerated startle response—palpitations
- Sleep disturbances
- Substance abuse
- Gastrointestinal disturbances

## Medications

### Antidepressants—Tricyclic
*Guide 203*
- Antidepressant
- Generic available
- Nonaddictive

### Benzodiazepines *Guide 210*
- Tranquilizer, anticonvulsant
- Generic available
- Addictive

### Buspirone (BuSpar) *Guide 214*
- Antianxiety
- Generic available
- Addictive

### SSRIs *Guide 249*
- Antidepressant, antiobsessional, antianxiety
- Some generics available
- Nonaddictive

### Venlafaxine (Effexor)
*Guide 255*
- Antidepressant—bicyclic
- No generic available
- Nonaddictive

## Assessment
- Assess scene safety *Guide 402*
- Use PPE *Guide 002*
- Approach patient *Guide 003*
- Primary and secondary medical survey *Guide 403*
- Medications and compliance
- Brief mental status exam *Guide 404*
- Brief psychosocial history *Guide 405*
- Emotional first aid *Guide 004*

## Reporting
- Description of patient
- Chief complaint
- Medical findings
- Medications and compliance
- Known diagnoses
- Mental status
- Psychosocial history

## GUIDE 131 SCHIZOPHRENIA

### Description
- Characterized by psychotic symptoms, including delusions or hallucinations, without patient having insight into their pathological nature

### Signs & Symptoms
- Delusions

- Hallucinations
- Disorganized speech
- Grossly disorganized or catatonic behavior
- Flat affect
- Alogia—poverty of speech
- Avolition—no motivation

### Paranoid Type

- Preoccupation with one or more delusions
- Auditory hallucinations

None of the following is prominent:

- Disorganized speech
- Disorganized behavior
- Catatonic behavior
- Flat affect
- Inappropriate affect

### Disorganized Type

- Disorganized speech
- Disorganized behavior
- Flat or inappropriate affect
- Echolalia—compulsive, senseless repetition of a word or phrase just spoken by another
- Echopraxia—pathological repetition of gestures made by others

### Catatonic Type

- Impaired motor functions
- Stupor
- Motionless
- Resistance to all instructions
- Rigid posture against attempts to move
- Voluntary posturing— voluntary assumptions of inappropriate or bizarre positions

### Residual Type

### Absence of the Following:

- Prominent delusions
- Hallucinations
- Disorganized speech
- Disorganized behavior
- Catatonic behavior

### Occurrence of the Following:

- Odd beliefs
- Unusual perceptual experiences
- Flat or inappropriate affect
- Alogia—poverty of speech
- Avolition—no motivation

## Medications

### Aripiprazole (Abilify)
*Guide 207*

- Antipsychotic
- No generic available
- Nonaddictive

### Carbamazepine (Tegretol)
*Guide 215*

- Analgesic, anticonvulsant, antimanic agent
- Generic available
- Nonaddictive

### Clozapine (Clozaril) *Guide 220*

- Antipsychotic
- Generic available
- Nonaddictive

### Haloperidol (Haldol)
Guide 226
- Antipsychotic
- Generic available
- Nonaddictive

### Loxapine Guide 230
- Tranquilizer, antidepressant
- Generic available
- Nonaddictive

### Molindone (Moban) Guide 237
- Antipsychotic
- No generic available
- Nonaddictive

### Olanzapine (Zyprexa)
Guide 241
- Antipsychotic
- No generic available
- Nonaddictive

### Phenothiazines Guide 245
- Tranquilizer, antiemetic
- Generic available
- Nonaddictive

### Quetiapine (Seroquel)
Guide 246
- Antipsychotic
- No generic available
- Nonaddictive

### Risperidone (Risperdal)
Guide 247
- Antipsychotic
- No generic available
- Nonaddictive

### Thiothixene Guide 251
- Antipsychotic
- Generic available
- Nonaddictive
- Correction of nerve impulses

## Assessment
- Assess scene safety Guide 402
- Use PPE Guide 002
- Approach patient Guide 003
- Primary and secondary medical survey Guide 403
- Medications
- Brief mental status exam Guide 404
- Brief psychosocial history Guide 405
- Emotional first aid Guide 004

## Reporting
- Description of patient
- Chief complaint
- Medical findings
- Medications and compliance
- Known diagnoses
- Mental status
- Psychosocial history

## Description

- Excessive anxiety concerning separation from home or from those to whom the patient is attached; onset before age 18
- Early onset—preschool, before age 6
- More common in girls than boys
- Genetics, temperament, stressful life events, and family can influence onset

## Signs & Symptoms

- Persistent, excessive distress when separated or anticipating separation
- Persistent, excessive worry about harm or loss of attachment figure
- Persistent reluctance to be alone
- Persistent reluctance or refusal to go to school or sleep away from home
- Repeated nightmares involving separation
- Patient complains of physical symptoms—headaches, nausea, or vomiting—when separation occurs

## Medications

*Antihistamines* Guide 205
- Antihistamine
- Generic available
- Nonaddictive

*Benzodiazepines* Guide 210
- Tranquilizer, anticonvulsant
- Generic available
- Addictive

*SSRIs* Guide 249
- Antidepressant, antiobsessional, antianxiety
- Some generics available
- Nonaddictive

## Assessment

- Assess scene safety *Guide 402*
- Use PPE *Guide 003*
- Approach patient *Guide 003*
- Primary and secondary medical survey *Guide 403*
- Medications and compliance
- Brief mental status exam *Guide 404*
- Brief psychosocial history *Guide 405*
- Emotional first aid *Guide 004*

## Reporting

- Description of patient
- Chief complaint
- Medical findings
- Medications and compliance
- Known diagnoses
- Mental status
- Psychosocial history

## Description

- Any type of unwanted or nonconsensual sexual activity
- All forms of sexual assaults are crimes

## Types of Sexual Assault

- Inappropriate touching
- Fondling
- Fellatio
- Cunnilingus
- Analingus
- Vaginal intercourse
- Anal intercourse
- Rape
- Attempted rape
- Child molestation *Guide 503*
- Incest *Guide 503*
- Voyeurism
- Exhibitionism
- Pornography
- Date rape drugs

### Some Common Date Rape Drugs

- Alcohol *Guide 302*
- Gamma hydroxybutyrate (GHB) *Guide 312*
- Ketamine *Guide 316*
- LSD *Guide 317*
- Rohypnol *Guide 326*

## Signs & Symptoms

### Physical

- The patient's report of sexual assault
- Bruising around the anus, breasts, or genital areas
- Torn, stained, or bloody underclothing
- Pregnancy
- Vaginal or anal bleeding
- Unexplained venereal disease or genital infection
- Black eye(s)
- Bone fractures
- Bruises
- Cuts
- Dislocations
- Internal injuries
- Lacerations
- Open wounds
- Punctures
- Rope marks
- Skull fractures
- Sprains

### Psychological

- Anger, rage
- Contradictory behavior
- Denial
- Depression
- Fear, terror
- Frenzied activity
- Frustration

1

- Grief and sorrow
- Guilt and self-blame
- Immobility
- Regression
- Screaming, crying, hysterical outbursts
- Self-destructive or other violent acts
- Shock, disbelief, confusion

## Survivor Care

- Ask if there is anyone you can help contact
- Avoid jargon, acronyms, codes, or other professional terminology
- Avoid judgments
- Be prepared to handle the grief reaction *Guide 117*
- Contact local sexual assault crisis center
- Do not jeopardize an ongoing investigation
- Maintain the chain of evidence and crime scene integrity—no shower, no bathroom; protect handprints and fingerprints
- Never leave the survivor(s) alone
- Relate the information in a calm, patient, and understanding manner

- Screen survivors from the media
- Stay until someone else arrives
- Try to put yourself in the survivor's place—have a caring attitude

## Assessment

- Assess scene safety *Guide 402*
- Use PPE *Guide 002*
- Approach patient *Guide 003*
- Primary and secondary medical survey *Guide 403*
- Medications and compliance
- Brief mental status exam *Guide 404*
- Lethality assessment *Guide 407*
- Emotional first aid *Guide 004*

## Reporting

- Description of patient
- Chief complaint
- Medical findings
- Medications and compliance
- Known diagnoses
- Mental status
- Lethality

## (GUIDE 134) SOMATIZATION DISORDER

### Description

- Chronic syndrome of physical complaints
- Cannot be explained medically
- More common in women than men

- Onset usually in adolescence or early adulthood
- Runs a fluctuating course with periods of remission and exacerbation

## Signs & Symptoms

- Can be represented by any organ or system
- Commonly expressed as neurological, gastrointestinal, psychosexual, or cardiopulmonary disorders

## Assessment

- Assess scene safety *Guide 402*
- Use PPE *Guide 002*
- Approach patient *Guide 003*
- Primary and secondary medical survey *Guide 403*
- Medications and compliance
- Brief mental status exam *Guide 404*
- Brief psychosocial history *Guide 405*
- Emotional first aid *Guide 004*

## Reporting

- Description of patient
- Chief complaint
- Medical findings
- Medications and compliance
- Known diagnoses
- Mental status
- Psychosocial history

1

## GUIDE 135 SUICIDE

## Description

- A self-inflicted death in which the patient acts intentionally, directly, and consciously
- An attempt to self-inflict death in which the patient acts intentionally, directly, and consciously

## Signs & Symptoms

*Children & Adolescents*

- Depression or other mood disorder
- Aggressive/disruptive behavior
- Substance abuse
- Sudden decline in school-work and/or attendance
- Withdrawal from social relationships
- Giving away prized possessions
- Running away
- Talking about death and/or suicide
- Attempted suicide

*Adults*

- Depression or other mood disorder
- Sudden mood swings

- Aggressive behavior
- Excessive risk-taking
- Personality change
- Social withdrawal
- Preoccupation with death
- Direct threats to commit suicide

*Elderly*
- Depression or other mood disorder
- Substance abuse
- Social withdrawal
- Preoccupation with death
- Putting business and legal affairs in order
- Changing of a will

## Risk Factors

*Children & Adolescents*
- Depression or other mood disorder
- Abuse—victimization
- Substance abuse
- Shame, humiliation, failure, or rejection
- Death of someone close—especially by suicide
- Family history of suicide
- Prior suicide attempt
- Access to a firearm

*Adults*
- Depression or other mood disorder
- Substance abuse
- Shame, humiliation, or failure
- Sudden rejection or unexpected separation
- Anticipated loss of financial security or personal freedom
- Chronic debilitating illness
- Diagnosis of a terminal illness
- Family history of suicide
- Prior suicide attempt
- Access to a firearm

*Elderly*
- Depression or other mood disorder
- Substance abuse
- Abuse—victimization
- Death of someone close—especially by suicide
- Sudden rejection or unexpected separation
- Anticipated loss of financial security or personal freedom
- Chronic debilitating illness
- Diagnosis of a terminal illness
- Family history of suicide
- Prior suicide attempt
- Access to a firearm

## Assessment

- Assess scene safety *Guide 402*
- Use PPE *Guide 002*
- Approach patient *Guide 003*
- Primary and secondary medical survey *Guide 403*
- Medications and compliance
- Brief mental status exam *Guide 404*

- Lethality assessment
  *Guide 407*
- Brief psychosocial history
  *Guide 405*
- Emotional first aid
  *Guide 004*

## Reporting

- Description of patient
- Chief complaint
- Medical findings
- Mental status
- Lethality
- Psychosocial history

## (GUIDE 136) TOURETTE'S DISORDER

### Description

- Recurrent motor and vocal tics
- Tics may occur many times throughout the day
- There is never a tic-free period of more than 3 months
- Tics are not the result of substance abuse or other medical condition

### Signs & Symptoms

- Repetitive, uncontrollable motor tics
- Motor tics usually involve the head and frequently other parts of the body
- Repetitive, uncontrollable vocal tics
- Vocal tics can include words or sounds such as grunts, clicks, snorts, barks, or coughs
- Coprolalia—complex vocal tic involving the utterance of obscenities

### Medications

*Antidyskinetics* Guide 204
- Antiparkinsonism
- Dopamine agonist
- Generic available
- Nonaddictive

*Clozapine (Clozaril)* Guide 220
- Antipsychotic
- Generic available
- Nonaddictive

*Haloperidol (Haldol)*
*Guide 226*
- Antipsychotic
- Generic available
- Nonaddictive

*Olanzapine (Zyprexa)*
*Guide 241*
- Antipsychotic
- No generic available
- Nonaddictive

*Risperidone (Risperdal)*
*Guide 247*
- Antipsychotic
- No generic available
- Nonaddictive

*SSRIs Guide 249*
- Antidepressant, antiobsessional, antianxiety
- Some generics available
- Nonaddictive

## Assessment

- Assess scene safety
  *Guide 402*
- Use PPE *Guide 002*
- Approach patient *Guide 003*
- Primary and secondary medical survey *Guide 403*
- Medications and compliance
- Brief mental status exam
  *Guide 404*

- Brief psychosocial history
  *Guide 405*
- Emotional first aid
  *Guide 004*

## Reporting

- Description of patient
- Chief complaint
- Medical findings
- Medications and compliance
- Known diagnoses
- Mental status
- Psychosocial history

## (GUIDE 137) TRAUMATIC BRAIN INJURY

### Description

- Presence of dementia as a consequence of head trauma
- Usually nonprogressive

### Signs & Symptoms

- Aphasia—confusion of words, inability to recall correct words
- Dysphasia—complete or partial loss of ability to understand, speak, read, and/or write
- Slurred speech
- Difficulty concentrating
- Irritability
- Anxiety
- Depression
- Mood swings

- Increased aggression
- Changes in personality

### Assessment

- Assess scene safety
  *Guide 402*
- Use PPE *Guide 002*
- Approach patient *Guide 003*
- Primary and secondary medical survey *Guide 403*
- Medications and compliance
- Brief mental status exam
  *Guide 404*
- Brief psychosocial history
  *Guide 405*
- Lethality assessment
  *Guide 407*
- Emotional first aid
  *Guide 004*

## Reporting

- Description of patient
- Chief complaint
- Medical findings
- Medications and compliance
- Known diagnoses
- Mental status
- Psychosocial history

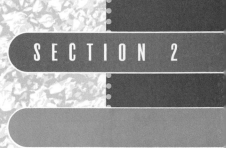

# SECTION 2

# Psychotropic Medications

# GUIDE 201 — PSYCHOTROPIC MEDICATIONS: ALPHABETICAL INDEX

| Medication | Guide No. | Page |
|---|---|---|
| Abilify | 207 | 87 |
| Acabamate | 233 | 119 |
| Acebutolol | 211 | 93 |
| Acetophenazine | 245 | 131 |
| Adapin | 203 | 82 |
| Adderall | 202 | 80 |
| Adderall XR | 202 | 80 |
| Advicor | 240 | 127 |
| Akineton | 204 | 84 |
| Allerdryl | 205 | 85 |
| AllerMax Caplets | 205 | 85 |
| Alprazolam | 210 | 91 |
| Alprazolam Intensol | 210 | 91 |
| Alurate | 209 | 89 |
| Amantadine | 206 | 86 |
| Amaphen | 209 | 89 |
| Ami Rax | 227 | 112 |
| Amitriptyline | 203 | 82 |
| Amobarbital | 209 | 89 |
| Amoxapine | 203 | 82 |
| Amphetamine | 202 | 80 |
| Amytal | 209 | 89 |
| Anafranil | 203 | 82 |
| Ancalixir | 209 | 89 |
| Anolor-300 | 209 | 89 |
| Anoquan | 209 | 89 |
| Antabuse | 221 | 105 |
| Anxanil | 227 | 112 |
| Apo-Alpraz | 210 | 91 |

| | | |
|---|---|---|
| Apo-Amitriptyline | 203 | **82** |
| Apo-Atenolol | 211 | **94** |
| Apo-Benztropine | 204 | **84** |
| Apo-Carbamazepine | 215 | **99** |
| Apo-Chlordiazepoxide | 210 | **91** |
| Apo-Clorazepate | 210 | **91** |
| Apo-Diazepam | 210 | **91** |
| Apo-Fluphenazine | 245 | **132** |
| Apo-Flurazepam | 210 | **91** |
| Apo-Haloperidol | 226 | **111** |
| Apo-Hydroxyzine | 227 | **112** |
| Apo-Imipramine | 203 | **82** |
| Apo-Lorazepam | 210 | **91** |
| Apo-Meprobamate | 233 | **120** |
| Apo-Metoprolol | 211 | **94** |
| Apo-Oxazepam | 210 | **91** |
| Apo-Perphenazine | 245 | **132** |
| Apo-Propranolol | 211 | **94** |
| Apo-Thioridazine | 245 | **132** |
| Apo-Timol | 211 | **94** |
| Apo-Trifluoperazine | 245 | **132** |
| Apo-Trihex | 204 | **84** |
| Apo-Trimip | 203 | **82** |
| Aprobarbital | 209 | **89** |
| Aquachloral | 217 | **101** |
| Arcet | 209 | **89** |
| Aricept | 218 | **102** |
| Aripiprazole | 207 | **87** |
| Artane | 204 | **84** |
| Artane Sequels | 204 | **84** |
| Asendin | 203 | **82** |
| Atarax | 227 | **112** |
| Atenolol | 211 | **93** |

2

2

| | | |
|---|---|---|
| Betaxin | 250 | **138** |
| Betaxolol | 211 | **93** |
| Betaxon | 211 | **94** |
| Bewon | 250 | **138** |
| Biamine | 250 | **138** |
| Biperiden | 204 | **83** |
| Bisoprolol | 211 | **93** |
| Blanex | 242 | **128** |
| Blocadren | 211 | **94** |
| Brexin | 205 | **85** |
| Bromazepam | 210 | **91** |
| Bronkolixir | 209 | **89** |
| Bronkotabs | 209 | **89** |
| Bucet | 209 | **89** |
| Bupropion | 213 | **96** |
| Buspirone | 214 | **98** |
| Busodium | 209 | **89** |
| BuSpar | 214 | **98** |
| Butabarbital | 209 | **89** |
| Butace | 209 | **89** |
| Butalan | 209 | **90** |
| Butalbital | 209 | **89** |
| Butalgen | 209 | **89** |
| Butisol | 209 | **90** |
| Cafergot PB | 209 | **90** |
| Calmylin #4 | 205 | **85** |
| Carbamazepine | 215 | **99** |
| Carbex | 248 | **135** |
| Carbidopa and Levodopa | 216 | **100** |
| Carbolith | 229 | **114** |
| Carteolol | 211 | **93** |
| Cartrol | 211 | **94** |
| Carvedilol | 211 | **93** |

2

2

| | | |
|---|---:|---:|
| Ezol | 209 | **89** |
| Femcet | 209 | **89** |
| Fenylhist | 205 | **85** |
| Fiorgen PF | 209 | **89** |
| Fioricet | 209 | **89** |
| Fiorinal | 209 | **89** |
| Fiormor | 209 | **89** |
| Flexagin | 242 | **128** |
| Flexoject | 242 | **128** |
| Flexon | 242 | **128** |
| Flumadine | 206 | **86** |
| Fluoxetine | 249 | **136** |
| Fluphenazine | 245 | **131** |
| Flurazepam | 210 | **91** |
| Fluvoxamine | 249 | **136** |
| Focalin | 234 | **121** |
| Fortabs | 209 | **89** |
| Fynex | 205 | **85** |
| G-1 | 209 | **89** |
| Gemonil | 209 | **89** |
| Genahist | 205 | **85** |
| Gen-D-Phen | 205 | **85** |
| Gerimal | 223 | **107** |
| Glantamine | 218 | **102** |
| Guanfacine | 225 | **110** |
| Halazepam | 210 | **91** |
| Haldol | 226 | **111** |
| Haldol Decanoate | 226 | **111** |
| Haldol LA | 226 | **111** |
| Haloperidol | 226 | **111** |
| Halperon | 226 | **111** |
| Hydergine | 223 | **107** |
| Hydergine LC | 223 | **107** |

2

| | | |
|---|---|---|
| Hydramine | 205 | **85** |
| Hydramyn | 205 | **85** |
| Hydril | 205 | **85** |
| Hydrophed | 227 | **112** |
| Hydroxyzine | 227 | **112** |
| Hyrexin-50 | 205 | **85** |
| Imipramine | 203 | **82** |
| Impril | 203 | **82** |
| Inderal | 211 | **94** |
| Inderal LA | 211 | **94** |
| Insomnal | 205 | **85** |
| Isobutal | 209 | **89** |
| Isocet | 209 | **89** |
| Isolin | 209 | **89** |
| Isollyl Improved | 209 | **89** |
| Isopap | 209 | **89** |
| Jumax | 248 | **135** |
| Jumexal | 248 | **135** |
| Juprenil | 248 | **135** |
| Kemadrin | 204 | **84** |
| Kerlone | 211 | **94** |
| Ketazolam | 210 | **91** |
| K-Flex | 242 | **128** |
| Klonopin | 210 | **91** |
| Labetalol | 211 | **93** |
| Laniroif | 209 | **89** |
| Lanorinal | 209 | **90** |
| Largactil | 245 | **132** |
| Largactil Liquid | 245 | **132** |
| Largactil Oral Drops | 245 | **132** |
| Larodopa | 228 | **113** |
| Lectopam | 210 | **91** |
| Leponex | 220 | **104** |

2

| | | |
|---|---|---|
| Marax | 227 | **112** |
| Marax DF | 227 | **112** |
| Marflex | 242 | **128** |
| Marnal | 209 | **90** |
| Mazepine | 215 | **99** |
| Mebaral | 209 | **90** |
| Medigesic | 209 | **90** |
| Medilium | 210 | **92** |
| Medi-Tran | 233 | **120** |
| Mellaril | 245 | **132** |
| Mellaril-S | 245 | **132** |
| Mephobarbital | 209 | **89** |
| Meprobamate | 233 | **119** |
| Meprospan 200 | 233 | **120** |
| Meprospan 400 | 233 | **120** |
| Mesoridazine | 245 | **132** |
| Metadate CD | 234 | **121** |
| Metadate ER | 234 | **121** |
| Methamphetamine | 202 | **80** |
| Metharbital | 209 | **89** |
| Methotrimeprazine | 245 | **132** |
| Methylin ER | 234 | **121** |
| Methylphenidate | 234 | **121** |
| Metoprolol | 211 | **94** |
| Meval | 210 | **92** |
| Midazolam | 210 | **91** |
| Miltown | 233 | **120** |
| Mirapex | 204 | **84** |
| Mirtazapine | 235 | **122** |
| Moban | 237 | **124** |
| Moban Concentrate | 237 | **124** |
| Modafinil | 236 | **123** |
| Modecate | 245 | **132** |

| | | |
|---|---|---|
| Modecate Concentrate | 245 | **132** |
| Moditen Enanthate | 245 | **132** |
| Moditen HCI | 245 | **132** |
| Moditen HCI-H.P. | 245 | **132** |
| Mogadon | 210 | **92** |
| Molindone | 237 | **124** |
| Monitan | 211 | **94** |
| Motion Aid | 205 | **85** |
| Movergan | 248 | **135** |
| Mudrane GG | 209 | **90** |
| Multipax | 227 | **112** |
| Myolin | 242 | **128** |
| Myotrol | 242 | **129** |
| Myproic Acid | 254 | **142** |
| Nadolol | 211 | **94** |
| Niacor | 240 | **127** |
| Naltrexone | 239 | **126** |
| Nardil | 231 | **117** |
| Navane | 251 | **139** |
| Nefazodone | 238 | **125** |
| Nembutal | 209 | **90** |
| Neocyten | 242 | **129** |
| Nervine Nighttime Sleep-Aid | 205 | **85** |
| Neuleptil | 245 | **132** |
| Neuramate | 233 | **120** |
| Nia-Bid | 240 | **127** |
| Niac | 240 | **127** |
| Niacels | 240 | **127** |
| Niacin | 240 | **127** |
| Nico-400 | 240 | **127** |
| Nicobid | 240 | **127** |
| Nicolar | 240 | **127** |
| Nicotinex | 240 | **127** |

| | | |
|---|---|---|
| Nicotinyl | 240 | **127** |
| Nidryl | 205 | **85** |
| Niloric | 223 | **107** |
| Nitrazepam | 210 | **91** |
| Noctec | 217 | **101** |
| Noradex | 242 | **129** |
| Noradryl | 205 | **85** |
| Norfranil | 203 | **82** |
| Normodyne | 211 | **94** |
| Norpramin | 203 | **82** |
| Nortriptyline | 203 | **82** |
| Nova-Rectal | 209 | **90** |
| Novo-Alprazol | 210 | **92** |
| Novo-Atenol | 211 | **94** |
| Novocarbamaz | 215 | **99** |
| Novochlorhydrate | 217 | **101** |
| Novo-Chlorpromazine | 245 | **132** |
| Novoclopate | 210 | **92** |
| Novodipam | 210 | **92** |
| Novo-Doxepin | 203 | **82** |
| Novoflupam | 210 | **92** |
| Novo-Flurazine | 245 | **132** |
| Novo-Hydroxyzin | 227 | **112** |
| Novolorazem | 210 | **92** |
| Novomepro | 233 | **120** |
| Novo-Mepro | 233 | **120** |
| Novometoprol | 211 | **94** |
| Novopentobarb | 209 | **90** |
| Novo-Peridol | 226 | **111** |
| Novo-Pindol | 211 | **94** |
| Novopoxide | 210 | **92** |
| Novopramine | 203 | **82** |
| Novopranol | 211 | **94** |

| | | |
|---|---|---|
| Novo-Ridazine | 245 | **132** |
| Novosecobarb | 209 | **90** |
| Novo-Timol | 211 | **94** |
| Novo-Tripramine | 203 | **82** |
| Novotriptyn | 203 | **82** |
| Novoxapam | 210 | **92** |
| Nozinan | 245 | **132** |
| Nozinan Liquid | 245 | **132** |
| Nozinan Oral Drops | 245 | **132** |
| Nu-Alpraz | 210 | **92** |
| Nu-Loraz | 210 | **92** |
| Nu-Metop | 211 | **94** |
| O-Flex | 242 | **129** |
| Olanzapine | 241 | **128** |
| Orap | 204 | **84** |
| Orflagen | 242 | **129** |
| Orfro | 242 | **129** |
| Orphenadrine | 242 | **128** |
| Orphenate | 242 | **129** |
| Oxazepam | 210 | **91** |
| Oxprenolol | 211 | **94** |
| Oxydess | 202 | **80** |
| Pacaps | 209 | **90** |
| Pamelor | 203 | **82** |
| Papulex | 240 | **127** |
| Parnate | 231 | **117** |
| Paroxetine | 249 | **136** |
| Parsidol | 204 | **84** |
| Parsitan | 204 | **84** |
| Pax 400 | 233 | **120** |
| Paxil | 249 | **136** |
| Paxil CR | 249 | **136** |
| Paxipam | 210 | **92** |

2

2

2

| | | |
|---|---|---|
| Ritalin SR | 234 | **121** |
| Rivastigmine | 218 | **102** |
| Rivotril | 210 | **92** |
| Ronigen | 240 | **127** |
| Roniacol | 240 | **127** |
| Ropinirole | 204 | **83** |
| Rycotin | 240 | **127** |
| Sarafem | 249 | **136** |
| Sarisol No. 2 | 209 | **90** |
| SD Deprenyl | 248 | **135** |
| Secobarbital | 209 | **89** |
| Secobarbital and Amobarbital | 209 | **89** |
| Seconal | 209 | **90** |
| Sectral | 211 | **94** |
| Sedabamate | 233 | **120** |
| Sedapap | 209 | **90** |
| Selegiline | 248 | **135** |
| Serax | 210 | **92** |
| Serentil | 245 | **132** |
| Serentil Concentrate | 245 | **132** |
| Seroquel | 246 | **133** |
| Sertraline | 249 | **136** |
| Serzone | 238 | **125** |
| Siladryl | 205 | **85** |
| Silphen | 205 | **85** |
| Simply Sleep | 205 | **85** |
| Sinemet | 216 | **100** |
| Sinemet-CR | 216 | **100** |
| Sinequan | 203 | **82** |
| Sleep-Eze | 205 | **85** |
| Slo-Niacin | 240 | **127** |
| Slow-Trasicor | 211 | **94** |
| Solazine | 245 | **132** |

| | | |
|---|---|---|
| Solfoton | 209 | **90** |
| Solium | 210 | **92** |
| Sominex Formula | 205 | **85** |
| Somnol | 210 | **92** |
| Sotacor | 211 | **94** |
| Sotalol | 211 | **94** |
| Spancap | 202 | **80** |
| Span-Niacin | 240 | **127** |
| Stelazine | 245 | **132** |
| Stelazine Concentrate | 245 | **132** |
| Stemetil | 245 | **132** |
| Stemetil Liquid | 245 | **132** |
| Strattera | 208 | **88** |
| Suprazine | 245 | **132** |
| Surmontil | 203 | **82** |
| Symadine | 206 | **86** |
| Symmetrel | 206 | **86** |
| Syn-Nadolol | 211 | **94** |
| Syn-Pindolol | 211 | **94** |
| Tacrine | 218 | **102** |
| Talbutal | 209 | **89** |
| Taro-Carbamazepine | 215 | **99** |
| Tasmar | 252 | **140** |
| Tecnal | 209 | **90** |
| Tega-Flex | 242 | **129** |
| Tega-Span | 240 | **127** |
| Tegretol | 215 | **99** |
| Tegretol Chewtabs | 215 | **99** |
| Tegretol CR | 215 | **99** |
| Temazepam | 210 | **91** |
| Tencet | 209 | **90** |
| Tenex | 225 | **110** |
| Tenormin | 211 | **94** |

2

| | | |
|---|---|---|
| Terfluzine | 245 | **132** |
| Terfluzine Concentrate | 245 | **132** |
| Theodrine | 209 | **90** |
| Theodrine Pediatric | 209 | **90** |
| Theofed | 209 | **90** |
| Thiamine (Vitamin B-1) | 250 | **138** |
| Thiopropazate | 245 | **131** |
| Thioproperazine | 245 | **131** |
| Thioridazine | 245 | **131** |
| Thiothixene | 251 | **138** |
| Thiothixene HCI Intensol | 251 | **139** |
| Thorazine | 245 | **132** |
| Thorazine Concentrate | 245 | **132** |
| Thorazine Spansule | 245 | **132** |
| Thor-Prom | 245 | **132** |
| Timolol | 211 | **94** |
| Tindal | 245 | **132** |
| Tofranil | 203 | **82** |
| Tofranil-PM | 203 | **82** |
| Tolcapone | 252 | **140** |
| Toprol | 211 | **94** |
| Toprol XL | 211 | **94** |
| Toprol XL-XR | 211 | **94** |
| T-Quil | 210 | **92** |
| Trancot | 233 | **120** |
| Trandate | 211 | **94** |
| Tranmep | 233 | **120** |
| Tranxene | 210 | **92** |
| Tranylcypromine | 231 | **116** |
| Tranxene T-Tab | 210 | **92** |
| Tranxene-SD | 210 | **92** |
| Trasicor | 211 | **94** |
| Trazodone | 253 | **141** |

| | | |
|---|---|---|
| Trazon | 253 | **141** |
| Triad | 209 | **90** |
| Triadapin | 203 | **82** |
| Trialodine | 253 | **141** |
| Triaprin | 209 | **90** |
| Triavil | 203 | **82** |
| Triavil | 245 | **132** |
| Tri-B3 | 240 | **127** |
| Trifluoperazine | 245 | **131** |
| Triflupromazine | 245 | **131** |
| Trihexane | 204 | **84** |
| Trihexy | 204 | **84** |
| Trihexyphenidyl | 204 | **83** |
| Trilafon | 245 | **132** |
| Trilafon Concentrate | 245 | **132** |
| Trimipramine | 203 | **82** |
| Tripramine | 203 | **82** |
| Triptil | 203 | **82** |
| Tuinal | 209 | **90** |
| Tusstat | 205 | **85** |
| Twilite | 205 | **85** |
| Two-Dyne | 209 | **90** |
| Ultrazine-10 | 245 | **132** |
| Unisom SleepGels Maximum Strength | 205 | **85** |
| Valium | 210 | **92** |
| Valproic Acid | 254 | **142** |
| Valrelease | 210 | **92** |
| Venlafaxine (Effexor) | 255 | **143** |
| Vesprin | 245 | **132** |
| Vibutal | 209 | **90** |
| Visken | 211 | **94** |
| Vistaril | 227 | **112** |
| Vivactil | 203 | **82** |

2

| | | |
|---|---|---|
| Vivol | 210 | **92** |
| Wehdryl-10 | 205 | **85** |
| Wehdryl-50 | 205 | **85** |
| Wellbutrin | 213 | **96** |
| Wellbutrin SR | 213 | **96** |
| Xanax | 210 | **92** |
| Zapex | 210 | **92** |
| Zebeta | 211 | **94** |
| Zebrax | 210 | **92** |
| Zetran | 210 | **92** |
| Zoloft | 249 | **136** |
| Zyban | 213 | **96** |
| Zyprexa | 241 | **128** |

## (GUIDE 202) AMPHETAMINES

### Description

- Central Nervous System (CNS) stimulant
- Generic available
- Addictive

### Generic & Brand Names

*Generic*

- Amphetamine
- Dextroamphetamine
- Methamphetamine

*Brand*

- Adderall
- Adderall XR
- Desoxyn
- Desoxyn Gradumet
- Dexedrine
- Dexedrine Spansule
- Oxydess
- Spancap

### Uses

- Attention Deficit Disorder (ADD)/Attention Deficit Hyperactivity Disorder (ADHD) *Guide 103*
- Depression in elderly patients *Guide 113*
- Narcolepsy *Guide 121*
- Short-term treatment for obesity

## Dosages

- Tablet
- Capsule, extended-release
- Tablet, extended-release

## Overdose Symptoms

- Tachycardia
- Hyperactivity
- Hyperthermia
- Hallucinations
- Suicidal or homicidal ideation *Guide 407*
- Seizures
- Coma

## Side Effects/Adverse Reactions

- Irritability
- Nervousness
- Insomnia
- Euphoria
- Dry mouth
- Tachycardia
- Headache
- Excess perspiration
- Weight loss
- Diminished sex drive
- Impotence

## Drug Interactions

### *Antihypertensives*

- Decreased antihypertensive effect

### *Beta-Blockers Guide 211*

- Hypertension
- Bradycardia

### *Carbonic Anhydrase Inhibitors*

- Increased amphetamine effect

### *Other CNS Stimulants*

- Excessive CNS stimulation

### *Furazolidone (Antibiotic)*

- Sudden and severe hypertension

### *Sympathomimetics*

- Seizures

### *Thyroid Hormones*

- Cardiac arrhythmias

## Other Interactions

### *Alcohol Guide 302*

- Decrcased amphetamine effect

### *Caffeine Drinks*

- Overstimulation

### *Cocaine Guide 307*

- Dangerous stimulation of the nervous system

### *Marijuana Guide 318*

- Frequent use—severely impaired mental function

2

## Description

- Antidepressants—Tricyclic
- Generic available
- Nonaddictive

## Generic & Brand Names

### *Generic*

- Amitriptyline
- Amoxapine
- Clomipramine
- Desipramine
- Doxepin
- Imipramine
- Nortriptyline
- Perphenazine and Amitriptyline
- Protriptyline
- Trimipramine

### *Brand*

- Adapin
- Anafranil
- Apo-Amitriptyline
- Apo-Imipramine
- Apo-Trimip
- Asendin
- Aventyl
- Elavil
- Elavil Plus
- Endep
- Etrafon
- Etrafon-A
- Etrafon-D
- Etrafon-F
- Etrafon-Forte
- Impril
- Levate
- Norfranil
- Norpramin
- Novo-Doxepin
- Novopramine
- Novo-Tripramine
- Novotriptyn
- Pamelor
- PMS Amitriptyline
- PMS Impramine
- PMS Levazine
- Rhotrimine
- Sinequan
- Surmontil
- Tofranil
- Tofranil-PM
- Triadapin
- Triavil
- Tripramine
- Triptil
- Vivactil

## Uses

- ADD/ADHD *Guide 103*
- Anxiety Disorder *Guide 106*
- Depression *Guide 113*
- Dissociative Identity Disorder *Guide 114*
- Bulimia *Guide 116*
- Narcolepsy *Guide 121*
- Obsessive Compulsive Disorder *Guide 122*
- Panic attacks *Guide 124*
- Post-Traumatic Stress Disorder (PTSD) *Guide 130*

- Cocaine withdrawal
  *Guide 307*
- Bed-wetting in children
- Pain relief

## Dosages

- Tablet
- Capsule
- Syrup

## Overdose Symptoms

- Hallucinations
- Drowsiness
- Dilated pupils
- Respiratory arrest
- Cardiac arrhythmias
- Convulsions
- Coma

## Side Effects/Adverse Reactions

- Headaches
- Dry mouth
- Constipation
- Diarrhea

- Nausea
- Fatigue
- Muscular weakness
- Nervousness, anxiety
- Insomnia

## Drug Interactions

*Andrenocorticoids—Systemic*

- Increased risk of mental side effects

*Anticoagulants—Oral*

- Possible increased anti-coagulant effect

## Other Interactions

*Alcohol*

- Increases intoxication

*Cocaine*

- Increases risk of cardiac arrhythmias

*Marijuana*

- Extreme drowsiness

# GUIDE 204 ANTIDYSKINETICS

## Description

- Antiparkinsonism
- Dopamine agonists
- Generic available
- Nonaddictive

## Generic & Brand Names

*Generic*

- Benztropine

- Biperiden
- Comtan
- Ethopropazine
- Pimozide
- Pramipexole
- Procyclidine
- Ropinirole
- Trihexyphenidyl

### Brand

- Akineton
- Apo-Benztropine
- Apo-Trihex
- Artane
- Artane Sequels
- Cogentin
- Comtan
- Kemadrin
- Mirapex
- Orap
- Parsidol
- Parsitan
- PMS Benztropine
- PMS Procyclidine
- PMS Trihexyphenidyl
- Procyclid
- Requip
- Trihexane
- Trihexy

## Uses

- Parkinson's Disease
  *Guide 126*
- Tourette's Disorder
  *Guide 136*
- Adverse effects of CNS drugs

## Dosages

- Tablet
- Extended-release capsule or liquid

## Overdose Symptoms

- Hallucinations
- Tachycardia
- Dilated pupils
- Drowsiness

## Side Effects/Adverse Reactions

- Blurred vision
- Sensitivity to light
- Incoordination
- Difficulty urinating

## Drug Interactions

*CNS Depressants*

- May increase sedation effects

## Other Interactions

*Alcohol Guide 302*

- Excessive sedation

---

## GUIDE 205   ANTIHISTAMINES

### Description

- Histamine blocker
- Generic available
- Nonaddictive

### Generic & Brand Names

*Generic*

- Diphenhydramine

### Brand

- Allerdryl
- AllerMax Caplets
- Banophen
- Banophen Caplets
- Beldin
- Belix
- Bena-D 10
- Bena-D 50
- Benadryl 25
- Benadryl Decongestant
- Benadryl Kapseals
- Benadryl Plus
- Benahist 10
- Benahist 50
- Ben-Allergin
- Benaphen
- Benoject-10
- Benoject-50
- Benylin Decongestant
- Brexin
- Calmylin #4
- Compoz
- Diphenacen-10
- Diphenacen-50
- Diphenadryl
- Dormarex 2
- Dormin
- Fenylhist
- Fynex
- Genahist
- Gen-D-phen
- Hydramine
- Hydramyn
- Hydril
- Hyrexin-50
- Insomnal
- Motion Aid
- Nervine Nighttime
  Sleep-Aid
- Nidryl
- Noradryl
- Nytol Maximum Strength
- Nytol with DPH
- Phendry
- Siladryl
- Silphen
- Simply Sleep
- Sleep-Eze
- Sominex Formula
- Tusstat
- Twilite
- Unisom SleepGels
  Maximum Strength
- Wehdryl-10
- Wehdryl-50

## Uses

- Alzheimer's Disease
  *Guide 104*
- Parkinson's Disease
  *Guide 126*
- Separation anxiety disorder
  *Guide 132*
- Sleep inducement
- Allergies
- Motion sickness
- Common cold

## Dosages

- Tablet
- Capsule
- Liquid

## Overdose Symptoms

- Flushed features
- Convulsions
- Coma

## Side Effects/Adverse Reactions

- Dry mouth, nose, throat
- Drowsiness
- Dizziness

## Drug Interactions

*Antidepressants*

- Increased sedation

*CNS Depressants*

- Increased sedation

*Dirithromycin*

- Serious cardiac arrhythmias

*Hypnotics*

- Increased sedation

*Molindone Guide 237*

- Sedation

*Narcotics*

- Heavy sedation

*Sedatives*

- Heavy sedation

*Sleep Inducers*

- Heavy sedation

*Tranquilizers*

- Heavy sedation

## Other Interactions

*Alcohol Guide 302*

- Increased sedation

*Marijuana Guide 318*

- Increased sedation

---

## GUIDE 206 ANTIVIRALS—INFLUENZA

### Description

- Antiviral, antiparkinsonism
- Generic available
- Nonaddictive

### Generic & Brand Names

*Generic*

- Amantadine
- Rimantadine

*Brand*

- Symadine
- Symmetrel
- Flumadine

### Uses

- Parkinson's Disease *Guide 126*
- Type A influenza virus infections

### Dosages

- Capsule
- Liquid

### Overdose Symptoms

- Cardiac arrhythmias
- Hypotension
- Convulsions

- Hallucinations
- Violent behavior
- Disorientation
- Slurred speech
- Rolling eyes

## Side Effects/Adverse Reactions

- Headache
- Difficulty concentrating
- Dizziness
- Lightheadedness
- Insomnia
- Nightmares

## Drug Interactions

*Antidepressants — Tricyclic Guide 203*

- With Amantadine: confusion, hallucinations, nightmares

*Antidyskinetics Guide 204*

- With Amantadine: confusion, hallucinations, nightmares

*Antihistamines Guide 205*

- With Amantadine: confusion, hallucinations, nightmares

## Other Interactions

*Alcohol Guide 302*

- Increases effects of alcohol

*Cocaine Guide 307*

- Dangerous overstimulation

2

---

## (GUIDE 207) ARIPIPRAZOLE (ABILIFY)

### Description

- Antipsychotic
- No generic available
- Nonaddictive
- Blocks certain impulses between nerve cells

### Generic & Brand Names

*Generic*

- Aripiprazole

*Brand*

- Abilify

### Uses

- Severe anxiety *Guide 106*
- Conduct Disorder *Guide 108*
- Paranoia *Guide 125*
- Schizophrenia *Guide 131*

### Dosages

- Tablet

## Overdose Symptoms

- Possible drowsiness
- Possible vomiting

## Side Effects/Adverse Reactions

- Hyperthermia
- Tachycardia
- Excessive perspiration

- Muscle rigidity
- Confusion
- Irritability
- Seizures

## Other Interactions

*Alcohol Guide 302*

- Increases sedative effects

---

## (GUIDE 208) ATOMOXETINE (STRATTERA)

## Description

- Selective norepinephrine reuptake inhibitor
- Generic not available
- Nonaddictive
- Appears to block a chemical neurotransmitter in the brain having to do with attention and activity

## Generic & Brand Names

*Generic*

- Atomoxetine

*Brand*

- Strattera

## Uses

- ADD/ADHD *Guide 103*

## Dosages

- Capsule form
- Do not open capsule

## Overdose Symptoms

- Confusion

- Agitation
- Cardiac arrhythmias
- Seizures

## Side Effects/Adverse Reactions

*Children*

- Appetite loss
- Mood swings
- Nausea—vomiting
- Dizziness

*Adults*

- Insomnia—infrequent
- Dry mouth
- Stomach pain
- Constipation
- Decreased sex drive
- Impotence

## Drug Interactions

*Monoamine Oxidase (MAO) Inhibitors Guide 231*

- Serious reactions, potentially fatal

*Beta-Blockers* Guide 211

- Increased risk of heart problems

*Bronchodilators*

- Increased risk of heart problems

## (GUIDE 209) BARBITURATES

### Description

- Antiseizure
- Generic available
- Addictive
- Partially blocks nerve impulses at nerve-cell connections

### Generic & Brand Names

*Generic*

- Amobarbital
- Aprobarbital
- Butabarbital
- Butalbital
- Mephobarbital
- Metharbital
- Pentobarbital
- Phenobarbital
- Secobarbital
- Secobarbital and Amobarbital
- Talbutal

*Brand*

- Alurate
- Amaphen
- Amytal
- Ancalixir
- Anolor-300
- Anoquan
- Arcet
- Axotal
- Azma Aid
- Bancap
- Barbita
- Bronkolixir
- Bronkotabs
- Bucet
- Busodium
- Butace
- Butalan
- Butalgen
- Butisol
- Cafergot PB
- Dolmar
- Endolor
- Esgic
- Esgic-Plus 4
- Ezol
- Femcet
- Fiorgen PF
- Fioricet
- Fiorinal
- Fiormor
- Fortabs
- G-1
- Gemonil
- Isobutal
- Isocet
- Isolin
- Isollyl Improved
- Isopap
- Laniroif

- Lanorinal
- Luminal
- Marnal
- Mebaral
- Medigesic
- Mudrane GG
- Nembutal
- Nova-Rectal
- Novopentobarb
- Novosecobarb
- Pacaps
- Phrenilin
- Phrenilin Forte
- Primatene "P" Formula
- Repan
- Sarisol No. 2
- Seconal
- Sedapap
- Solfoton
- Tecnal
- Tencet
- Theodrine
- Theodrine Pediatric
- Theofed
- Triad
- Triaprin
- Tuinal
- Two-Dyne
- Vibutal

## Uses

- Anxiety Disorders
  *Guide 106*
- Epilepsy
- Prevention of febrile
  seizures
- Sleep aid—short-term basis
- Asthma
- Gastrointestinal disorders—
  in combination with other
  medicines

- Headaches—in combina-
  tion with other medicines
- Traumatic Brain Injury
  *Guide 137*

## Dosages

- Capsule
- Elixir
- Tablet
- Rectal suppository

## Overdose Symptoms

- Deep sleep
- Difficulty breathing
- Weak pulse
- Coma

## Side Effects/Adverse Reactions

- Dizziness
- Drowsiness
- Incoordination
- Confusion
- Headache
- Irritability
- Fainting
- Nausea—vomiting
- Depression
- Nightmares
- Difficulty sleeping

## Drug Interactions

*Anticonvulsants*

- Seizure pattern changes

*Antihistamines Guide 205*

- Dangerous sedation

### Carteolol

- Increased barbiturate effect—dangerous sedation

### Clozapine *Guide 220*

- Effects can be toxic to CNS

## Other Interactions

### Alcohol *Guide 302*

- Potentially fatal oversedation

### Cocaine *Guide 307*

- Decreased barbiturate effect

### Marijuana *Guide 318*

- Excessive sedation

---

## (GUIDE 210) BENZODIAZEPINES

### Description

- Tranquilizer
- Anticonvulsant
- Generic available
- Addictive

### Generic & Brand Names

*Generic*

- Alprazolam
- Bromazepam
- Chlordiazepoxide
- Clonazepam
- Clorazepate
- Diazepam
- Estrazolam
- Flurazepam
- Halazepam
- Ketazolam
- Lorazepam
- Midazolam
- Nitrazepam
- Oxazepam
- Prazepam
- Quazepam
- Temazepam

*Brand*

- Alprazolam Intensol
- Apo-Alpraz
- Apo-Chlordiazepoxide
- Apo-Clorazepate
- Apo-Diazepam
- Apo-Flurazepam
- Apo-Lorazepam
- Apo-Oxazepam
- Ativan
- Centrax
- Clindex
- Clinoxide
- Dalmane
- Diastat
- Diazemuls
- Diazepam Intensol
- Doral
- Klonopin
- Lectopam
- Librax

- Libritabs
- Librium
- Lidoxide
- Limbitrol
- Limbitrol DS
- Lipoxide
- Loftran
- Lorazepam Intensol
- Medilium
- Meval
- Mogadon
- Novo-Alprazol
- Novoclopate
- Novodipam
- Novoflupam
- Novolorazem
- Novopoxide
- Novoxapam
- Nu-Alpraz
- Nu-Loraz
- Paxipam
- PMS Diazepam
- ProSom
- Restoril
- Rivotril
- Serax
- Solium
- Somnol
- T-Quil
- Tranxene
- Tranxene T-Tab
- Tranxene-SD
- Valium
- Valrelease
- Vivol
- Xanax
- Zapex
- Zebrax
- Zetran

## Uses

- Anxiety Disorders *Guide 106*
- Dissociative identity disorder *Guide 114*
- Obsessive compulsive disorder *Guide 122*
- Panic disorders *Guide 124*
- Personality disorders *Guide 127*
- Phobias *Guide 129*
- PTSD *Guide 130*
- Separation anxiety disorder *Guide 132*
- Alcohol withdrawal *Guide 302*
- Muscle spasms
- Seizure disorders
- Short-term insomnia
- Traumatic Brain Injury *Guide 137*

## Dosages

- Tablet
- Capsule
- Extended release capsule
- Oral suspension
- Sublingual tablet
- Rectal gel

## Overdose Symptoms

- Drowsiness
- Weakness
- Tremors
- Coma

## Side Effects/Adverse Reactions

- Drowsiness
- Dizziness

- Hallucinations
- Constipation

## Drug Interactions

### *Anticonvulsants*

- Change in seizure pattern

### *Antidepressants — Tricyclic* Guide 203

- Increased sedative effect, both drugs

### *Antihistamines* Guide 205

- Increased sedative effect, both drugs

### *CNS Depressants*

- Increased sedative effect

### *MAO Inhibitors* Guide 231

- Seizures

- Deep sedation
- Rage

## Other Interactions

### *Alcohol* Guide 302

- Heavy sedation

### *Cocaine* Guide 307

- Decreased benzodiazepine effect

### *Marijuana* Guide 318

- Heavy sedation

### *Tobacco*

- Decreased benzodiazepine effect

---

## (GUIDE 211) BETA-BLOCKERS

### Description

- Beta-Adrenergic Blocking Agents
- Antiadrenergic, antianginal, antiarrhythmic, antihypertensive
- Generic available
- Nonaddictive
- Diuretic: forces sodium and water excretion and relaxes muscle cells of small arteries

### Generic & Brand Names

#### *Generic*

- Acebutolol
- Atenolol
- Betaxolol
- Bisoprolol
- Carteolol
- Carvedilol
- Labetalol
- Levobetaxolol

- Metoprolol
- Nadolol
- Oxprenolol
- Penbutolol
- Pindolol
- Propranolol
- Sotalol
- Timolol

*Brand*

- Apo-Atenol
- Apo-Metoprolol
- Apo-Propranolol
- Apo-Timol
- Betaloc
- Betapace
- Betaxon
- Blocadren
- Cartrol
- Coreg
- Corgard
- Detensol
- Inderal
- Inderal LA
- Kerlone
- Levatol
- Lopressor
- Lopressor SR
- Monitan
- Normodyne
- Novo-Atenol
- Novometoprol
- Novo-Pindol
- Novopranol
- Novo-Timol
- Nu-Metop
- Sectral
- Slow-Trasicor
- Sotacor

- Syn-Nadolol
- Syn-Pindolol
- Tenormin
- Toprol
- Toprol XL
- Toprol XL-XR
- Trandate
- Trasicor
- Visken
- Zebeta

## Uses

- Anxiety Disorders *Guide 106*
- Alcoholism *Guide 302*
- Hypertension
- Edema
- Angina
- Stabilizes cardiac arrhythmias
- Hypertension
- Decreases frequency of migraine headaches

## Dosages

- Extended-release capsules

## Overdose Symptoms

- Cardiac arrhythmia
- Bradycardia
- Seizures
- Confusion
- Fainting
- Convulsions
- Coma

## Side Effects/Adverse Reactions

- Wheezing
- Chest pain

- Cardiac arrhythmia
- Dry mouth
- Weak pulse
- Nausea—vomiting
- Muscle cramping
- Mood swings
- Insomnia
- Constipation
- Depression

## Drug Interactions

### Allopurinol

- Decreases allopurinol effect

### Aminophylline

- Decreases effectiveness of both

### Antidepressants—Tricyclic
Guide 203

- Dangerous hypotension

## Other Interactions

### Alcohol Guide 302

- Dangerous hypotension

### Cocaine Guide 307

- Cardiac arrhythmias; decreases beta-blocker effect

### Licorice

- Excessive potassium loss, leading to dangerous heart rhythms

### Marijuana Guide 318

- Possible hypertension
- Tobacco
- Possible hypertension
- Forces heart to work harder

2

---

# (GUIDE 212) BROMOCRIPTINE

## Description

- Antiparkinsonism
- Generic available
- Nonaddictive

## Generic & Brand Names

### Generic

- Bromocriptine

### Brand

- Alti-Bromocriptine
- Apo-Bromocriptine
- Parlodel
- Parlodel Snaptabs

## Uses

- Parkinson's Disease Guide 126
- Infertility
- Acromegaly—overproduction of growth hormone
- Pituitary tumors
- Sexual dysfunctions

## Dosages

- Tablet
- Capsule

## Overdose Symptoms

- Muscular twitches
- Spastic eye closure
- Nausea—vomiting
- Irregular and rapid pulse
- Fainting
- Disorientation
- Hallucinations
- Coma

## Side Effects/Adverse Reactions

- Dizziness
- Nausea
- Headache

## Drug Interactions

*Antihypertensives*

- Hypotension

*Ergot Alkaloids*

- Hypertension

## Other Interactions

*Alcohol Guide 302*

- Decreased alcohol tolerance

*Marijuana Guide 318*

- Increases fatigue
- Lethargy
- Fainting

---

## (GUIDE 213) BUPROPION

## Description

- Antidepressant
- No generic available
- Nonaddictive

## Generic & Brand Names

*Generic*

- Bupropion

*Brand*

- Wellbutrin
- Wellbutrin SR
- Zyban

## Uses

- ADD/ADHD *Guide 103*
- Depression *Guide 113*
- PTSD *Guide 130*
- Smoking cessation

## Dosages

- Tablet

## Overdose Symptoms

- Confusion
- Agitation
- Seizures
- Coma

## Side Effects/Adverse Reactions

- Excitement
- Anxiety
- Insomnia
- Restlessness
- Constipation
- Appetite suppression

- Dry mouth
- Dizziness
- Nausea or vomiting
- Confusion
- Cardiac arrhythmia
- Severe headache
- Seizure

## Drug Interactions

*Antidepressants — Tricyclic*
*Guide 203*

- Increased risk of seizures

*Carbamazepine* *Guide 215*

- Risk of seizures

*Clozapine* *Guide 220*

- Increased risk of seizures

*Fluoxetine* *Guide 249*

- Increased risk of seizures

*Haloperidol* *Guide 226*

- Increased risk of seizures

*Lithium* *Guide 229*

- Increased risk of seizures

*Loxapine* *Guide 230*

- Increased risk of seizures

*Maprotiline* *Guide 232*

- Increased risk of seizures

*Molindone* *Guide 237*

- Increased risk of seizures

*MAO Inhibitors* *Guide 231*

- Increased risk of seizures

*Phenothiazines* *Guide 245*

- Increased risk of seizures

*Phenytoin*

- Increased risk of seizures

*Thiothixene* *Guide 251*

- Increased risk of seizures

*Trazodone* *Guide 253*

- Increased risk of seizures

## Other Interactions

*Alcohol* *Guide 302*

- Increased risk of seizures

*Beverages: Coffee, Tea, Cocoa*

- Restlessness and insomnia

*Cocaine* *Guide 307*

- Increased risk of seizures

*Marijuana* *Guide 318*

- Increased risk of seizures

**2**

## (GUIDE 214) BUSPIRONE

### Description
- Antianxiety agent
- Generic available
- Nonaddictive

### Generic & Brand Names

*Generic*
- Buspirone

*Brand*
- BuSpar

### Uses
- Chronic Anxiety Disorder *Guide 106*
- Dementia *Guide 112*
- Dissociative Identity Disorder *Guide 114*
- Obsessive Compulsive Disorder *Guide 122*
- Phobias *Guide 129*
- Anxiety in alcoholics or substance abusers *Guide 302*

### Dosages
- Tablets—take with food

### Overdose Symptoms
- Severe drowsiness
- Nausea—vomiting
- Constricted pupils
- Unconsciousness

### Side Effects/Adverse Reactions
- Chest pain
- Tachycardia
- Lightheadedness
- Dizziness
- Nausea
- Fatigue
- Drowsiness
- Ringing in ears
- Nightmares

### Drug Interactions

*Barbiturates Guide 209*
- Excessive sedation

*CNS Depressants*
- Increased sedative effect

*MAO Inhibitors Guide 231*
- Possible hypertension

*Narcotics*
- Excessive synergistic effects

### Other Interactions

*Alcohol Guide 302*
- Excessive sedation

*Caffeine*
- Decreases antianxiety effect of Buspirone

*Marijuana Guide 318*
- Decreases antianxiety effect of Buspirone

*Tobacco*
- Decreases antianxiety effect of Buspirone

## Description

- Analgesic
- Anticonvulsant
- Antimanic agent
- Generic available
- Nonaddictive
- Reduces excitability of nerve fibers in brain; reduces transmission of pain messages at certain nerve terminals

## Generic & Brand Names

### Generic

- Carbamazepine

### Brand

- Apo-Carbamazepine
- Epitol
- Mazepine
- Novocarbamaz
- PMS Carbamazepine
- Taro-Carbamazepine
- Tegretol
- Tegretol Chewtabs
- Tegretol CR

## Uses

- Bipolar Disorder *Guide 107*
- Conduct Disorder *Guide 108*
- Paranoia *Guide 125*
- Schizophrenia *Guide 131*
- Alcohol withdrawal *Guide 302*
- Decreases severity and lengths of tics
- Prevents seizures
- Pain relief
- Traumatic Brain Injury *Guide 137*

## Dosages

- Regular tablet
- Chewable tablet

## Overdose Symptoms

- Uncontrollable movements
- Drowsiness
- Cardiac arrhythmia
- Decreased urination
- Hypotension
- Dilated pupils
- Flushed skin
- Coma

## Side Effects/Adverse Reactions

- Blurred vision
- Nystagmus (jerky eye movements)
- Confusion
- Slurred speech
- Fainting
- Depression
- Sore throat
- Fever

## Drug Interactions

### Adrenocorticoids

- Decreased effect of adreno-corticoid

### Anticoagulants

- Decreased anticoagulant effect

### Anticonvulsants
- Decreased effect of both

### Antidepressants—Tricyclic Guide 203
- Confusion
- Possible psychosis

### Bupropion Guide 213
- Seizure risk

### Clozapine Guide 220
- Toxic effect on bone marrow and CNS

### Digitalis Glycosides
- Excessive bradycardia

### MAO Inhibitors Guide 231
- Dangerous overstimulation

### Meglitinides
- Blood sugar problems

## Other Interactions

### Alcohol Guide 302
- Increased sedative effect of alcohol

### Cocaine Guide 307
- Increased adverse effects of Carbamazepine

### Marijuana Guide 318
- Increased adverse effects of Carbamazepine

---

## GUIDE 216 — CARBIDOPA & LEVODOPA

### Description
- Antiparkinsonism
- Generic available
- Nonaddictive
- Restores chemical balance, creating normal nerve impulses

### Generic & Brand Names

#### Generic
- Carbidopa and Levodopa

#### Brand
- Sinemet
- Sinemet-CR

### Use
- Parkinson's Disease Guide 126

### Dosage
- Tablet

### Overdose Symptoms
- Muscular twitching
- Spastic eyelid closure
- Agitation
- Nausea—vomiting
- Hallucinations
- Disorientation
- Fainting
- Coma
- Hypertension

## Side Effects/Adverse Reactions

- Mood swings
- Uncontrollable body movements
- Diarrhea
- Dry mouth
- Body odor

## Drug Interactions

### Antidepressants

- Weakness or faintness when getting up

### Antihypertensives

- Possible hypotension

### MAO Inhibitors Guide 231

- Can create dangerous hypertension

## Other Interactions

### Cocaine Guide 307

- Can increase cardiac arrhythmia

### Marijuana Guide 318

- Increased lethargy
- Fatigue
- Fainting

2

---

## GUIDE 217 — CHLORAL HYDRATE

### Description

- Sedative—hypnotic agent
- Generic available
- Addictive

### Generic & Brand Names

#### Generic

- Chloral hydrate

#### Brand

- Aquachloral
- Noctec
- Novochlorhydrate

### Use

- Insomnia

### Dosages

- Capsule
- Syrup
- Suppository

### Overdose Symptoms

- Confusion
- Weakness
- Difficulty breathing
- Jaundice
- Stupor
- Cardiac arrhythmia
- Loss of consciousness
- Seizures
- Coma

## Side Effects/Adverse Reactions

- Nausea and vomiting
- Stomach pain
- Incoordination
- Dizziness
- Drowsiness
- Light headedness
- Confusion
- Agitation
- Hallucinations

## Drug Interactions

*Anticoagulants*

- Possible hemorrhaging

*Antihypertensives*

- Excessive hypotension

*Clozapine Guide 220*

- Toxic effect on CNS

## Other Interactions

*Alcohol Guide 302*

- Increased sedation

*Marijuana Guide 318*

- Severe impairment of physical and mental functioning

---

**GUIDE 218** CHOLINESTERASE INHIBITORS

## Description

- Cholinesterase inhibitor
- Generic not available
- Nonaddictive
- Decreases breakdown of brain chemical acetylcholine

## Generic & Brand Names

*Generic*

- Donepezil
- Glantamine
- Rivastigmine
- Tacrine

*Brand*

- Aricept
- Razadyne
- Exelon
- Cognex

## Uses

- Alzheimer's Disease *Guide 104*
- Dementia *Guide 112*

## Dosages

- Capsule
- Tablet
- Liquid

## Overdose Symptoms

- Excessive saliva
- Severe nausea—vomiting
- Hypotension
- Bradycardia
- Muscle weakness

- Difficulty breathing
- Seizures

## Side Effects/Adverse Reactions

- Nausea—vomiting
- Diarrhea
- Incoordination

## Drug Interactions

### *Anticholinergics*

- Decreased anticholinergic effect

### *Antiinflammatories, Nonsteroidal*

- Can increase gastric acid secretions

---

## ( GUIDE 219 ) CLONIDINE

### Description

- Antihypertensive
- Generic available
- Nonaddictive

### Generic & Brand Names

#### *Generic*

- Clonidine

#### *Brand*

- Catapres
- Catapres-TTS
- Dixarit

### Uses

- Narcotic withdrawal syndrome
- Nicotine withdrawal
- Prevention of migraine headaches
- Controls overactivity and tics in children
- Hypertension

### Dosages

- Tablet
- Transdermal patch

### Overdose Symptoms

- Vomiting
- Fainting
- Bradycardia
- Chills
- Fatigue
- Shortness of breath
- Dizziness
- Diminished reflexes
- Coma

### Side Effects/Adverse Reactions

- Dizziness
- Constipation
- Drowsiness
- Dry mouth
- Fatigue
- Headache
- Depression

- Light-headedness
- Nausea and vomiting
- Burning eyes
- Nervousness
- Rebound hypertension upon rapid withdrawal

## Drug Interactions

*Antihypertensives*

- Excessive hypotension

*Beta-Blockers Guide 211*

- Sudden hypotension

## Other Interactions

*Alcohol Guide 302*

- Excessive hypotension
- Increased sedation

*Cocaine Guide 307*

- Hypertension
- Increased risk of heart block

*Marijuana Guide 318*

- Weakness upon standing

# (GUIDE 220) CLOZAPINE

## Description

- Antipsychotic
- Generic available
- Nonaddictive
- Dopamine inhibitor

## Generic & Brand Names

*Generic*

- Clozapine

*Brand*

- Clozaril
- Leponex

## Uses

- Conduct Disorder *Guide 108*
- Paranoia *Guide 125*
- Schizophrenia *Guide 131*
- Suicide reduction in patients with psychotic disorders *Guide 135*
- Tourette's Disorder *Guide 136*

## Dosages

- Tablet

## Overdose Symptoms

- Tachycardia
- Bradycardia
- Cardiac arrhythmias
- Hallucinations
- Difficulty breathing
- Drowsiness
- Excitement
- Restlessness

## Side Effects/Adverse Reactions

- High fever
- Rapid pulse
- Profuse sweating
- Muscular rigidity
- Confusion

- Irritability
- Seizures
- Chills

## Drug Interactions

*Antihypertensives*

- Serious hypotension

*Bupropion* Guide 213

- Increases risk of seizures

*CNS Depressants*

- Toxic to CNS

*Fluvoxamine* Guide 249

- Increases risk of seizures

*Haloperidol* Guide 226

- Increases risk of seizures

*Lithium* Guide 229

- Increases risk of seizures

## Other Interactions

*Alcohol* Guide 302

- Toxic to CNS

*Caffeine*

- Cardiac arrhythmia

*Cocaine* Guide 307

- Possible cardiac arrhythmia

*Marijuana* Guide 318

- Possible cardiac arrhythmia

2

# GUIDE 221 DISULFIRAM

## Description

- No drug class
- Generic available
- Nonaddictive
- When taken in combination with alcohol, produces a metabolic change that creates short-term toxicity

## Generic & Brand Names

*Generic*

- Disulfiram

*Brand*

- Antabuse

## Use

- Alcoholism *Guide 302*

## Dosage

- Tablet

## Overdose Symptoms

- Memory loss
- Behavior disturbances
- Lethargy
- Confusion
- Headaches
- Nausea—vomiting
- Stomach pain
- Diarrhea

- Weakness
- Temporary paralysis

## Side Effects/Adverse Reactions

- Drowsiness
- Eye pain
- Vision change
- Stomach discomfort
- Headache
- Mood change
- Decreased sexual ability

## Drug Interactions

*Anticoagulants*

- Possible unexplained bleeding

*Anticonvulsants*

- Excessive sedation

*Barbiturates Guide 209*

- Excessive sedation

*CNS Depressants*

- Increased depressive effect

*Clozapine Guide 220*

- Toxic effect on the CNS

## Other Interactions

*Alcohol Guide 302*

- Potentially fatal toxicity

*Cocaine Guide 307*

- Increased Disulfiram effect

*Foods Prepared with Alcohol*

- Causes Disulfiram effect

*Some Foods Prepared with Alcohol*

- Sauces
- Fermented vinegar
- Marinades
- Desserts

---

## GUIDE 222 DIVALPROEX

### Description

- Anticonvulsant
- No generic available
- Nonaddictive
- Increases gamma amino-butyric acid—inhibits nerve transmission in parts of the brain

### Brand Names

- Depakote
- Depakote Sprinkle
- Epival

### Uses

- Bipolar Disorder—treats the manic phase *Guide 107*
- Conduct Disorder *Guide 108*
- Epilepsy—controls petit mal seizures
- Migraine headaches
- Traumatic Brain Injury *Guide 137*

### Dosages

- Delayed-release capsule
- Delayed-release liquid
- Sprinkle

## Overdose Symptom

- Coma

## Side Effects/Adverse Reactions

- Loss of appetite
- Indigestion
- Nausea or vomiting
- Poor coordination
- Diarrhea
- Weight gain/loss
- Stomach cramps

## Drug Interactions

### Anticoagulants

- Increased chance of bleeding

### Aspirin

- Increased risk of bleeding

### CNS Depressants

- Increased sedation

### Clonazepam *Guide 210*

- May cause or prolong seizure

### MAO Inhibitors *Guide 231*

- Increased sedation

## Other Interactions

### Alcohol *Guide 302*

- Deep sedation

### Cocaine *Guide 307*

- Increases brain sensitivity

### Marijuana *Guide 318*

- Increases brain sensitivity

### Tobacco

- Increases brain sensitivity

2

---

# (GUIDE 223) ERGOLOID MESYLATES

## Description

- Ergot preparation
- Generic available
- Nonaddictive

## Generic & Brand Names

### Generic

- Ergoloid mesylates

### Brand

- Gerimal
- Hydergine
- Hydergine LC
- Niloric

## Uses

- Dementia *Guide 112*
- Depression—elderly patients *Guide 113*

## Dosages

- Tablet
- Sublingual tablet
- Capsule
- Liquid

## Overdose Symptoms

- Headache
- Flushed features
- Nasal congestion
- Nausea—vomiting
- Blurred vision
- Weakness
- Collapse
- Coma

## Side Effects/Adverse Reactions

- Runny nose
- Flushed features
- Headache
- Bradycardia

## Drug Interactions

### *Other Ergot Preparations*

- Decreased circulation to extremities

## Other Interactions

### *Alcohol Guide 302*

- May cause hypotension

### *Cocaine Guide 307*

- Overstimulation

### *Marijuana Guide 318*

- Decreased effect of ergot alkaloids

### *Tobacco*

- Decreased ergoloid effect

---

## GUIDE 224 — ERGOTAMINE, BELLADONNA, & PHENOBARBITAL

## Description

- Analgesic, antispasmodic, vasoconstrictor
- No generic available
- Addictive

## Generic & Brand Names

### *Generic*

- Ergotamine, belladonna, phenobarbital

### *Brand*

- Bellergal
- Bellergal-S
- Bellergal Spacetabs

## Uses

- Anxiety Disorder *Guide 106*
- Vascular headaches
- Nervous tension
- Menopause

## Dosages

- Tablet
- Extended-release tablet

## Overdose Symptoms

- Tingling
- Cold extremities
- Numbness in extremities
- Muscle pain
- Nausea—vomiting
- Dilated pupils
- Tachycardia
- Rapid breathing
- Confusion
- Slurred speech
- Agitation
- Flushed features
- Convulsions
- Coma

## Side Effects/Adverse Reactions

- Flushed skin
- Fever
- Drowsiness
- Bloating
- Depression *Guide 113*
- Frequent urination
- Constipation
- Dizziness
- Increased severity and frequency of headaches
- "Hangover" effects

## Drug Interactions

*Amphetamines* Guide 202

- Dangerous hypertension

*Anticonvulsants*

- Changes in seizure patterns

*Antihistamines* Guide 205

- Severe and dangerous sedation

*Beta-Blockers* Guide 211

- Narrowing of the arteries in heart if taken in large doses

## Other Interactions

*Alcohol* Guide 302

- Potential fatal oversedation

*Amphetamines* Guide 303

- Dangerous hypertension

*Cocaine* Guide 307

- Excessive tachycardia

*Marijuana* Guide 318

- Drowsiness
- Dry mouth
- Oversedation

2

## GUIDE 225 — GUANFACINE

### Description

- Antihypertensive
- No generic available
- Nonaddictive

### Generic & Brand Names

*Generic*

- Guanfacine

*Brand*

- Tenex

### Uses

- Controls overactivity and tics in children
- Hypertension

### Dosages

- Tablet

### Overdose Symptoms

- Difficulty breathing
- Dizziness
- Bradycardia
- Loss of consciousness

### Side Effects/Adverse Reactions

- Constipation
- Dry mouth
- Confusion
- Dizziness
- Drowsiness
- Fainting
- Headache
- Movement disorders
- Depression
- Bradycardia
- Nausea and vomiting
- Burning eyes

### Drug Interactions

*Antihypertensives*

- Excessive hypotension

*Carteolol*

- Increased hypotension

*CNS Depressants*

- Increased depressant effect

*Clozapine Guide 220*

- Toxic effect on CNS

*Methyprylon*

- Dangerous sedation

*Nicardipine*

- Sudden hypotension

*Nimodipine*

- Dangerous hypotension

### Other Interactions

*Alcohol Guide 302*

- Excess use may lead to dangerous hypotension

*Cocaine Guide 307*

- Hypertension
- Increased risk of heart block

## (GUIDE 226) HALOPERIDOL

### Description

- Dopamine blocker
- Generic available
- Nonaddictive
- Corrects imbalance in nerve impulses from brain

### Generic & Brand Names

*Generic*

- Haloperidol

*Brand*

- Apo-Haloperidol
- Haldol
- Haldol Decanoate
- Haldol LA
- Halperon
- Novo-Peridol
- Peridol
- PMS Haloperidol

### Uses

- Severe anxiety *Guide 106*
- Conduct Disorder *Guide 108*
- Dementia *Guide 112*
- Paranoia *Guide 125*
- Schizophrenia *Guide 131*
- Tourette's Disorder *Guide 136*
- Infantile autism
- Huntington's chorea

### Dosages

- Tablet
- Drops—concentrated

### Overdose Symptoms

- Weak pulse
- Tachycardia
- Slow and shallow respirations
- Extreme hypotension
- Muscle weakness
- Muscular tremors
- Convulsions
- Deep sleep, ending in coma

### Side Effects/Adverse Reactions

- High fever
- Tachycardia
- Increased perspiration
- Confusion
- Muscle rigidity
- Confusion
- Irritability
- Seizures
- Movement disorders

### Drug Interactions

*Anticonvulsants*

- Changes in seizure pattern

*Antidepressants*

- Excessive sedation

*Barbiturates Guide 209*

- Excessive sedation

*Bupropion Guide 213*

- Increased risk of seizures

### CNS Depressants

- Increases CNS depression
- Hypotension

### Clozapine *Guide 220*

- Toxic effects on the nervous system

## Other Interactions

### Alcohol *Guide 302*

- Deep sedation
- Decreased brain function

### Cocaine *Guide 307*

- Decreases effect of haloperidol

### Marijuana *Guide 318*

- Frequent use may result in toxic psychosis

---

# GUIDE 227  HYDROXYZINE

## Description

- Antianxiety
- Generic available
- Nonaddictive
- Histamine blocker

## Generic & Brand Names

### Generic

- Hydroxyzine

### Brand

- Ami Rax
- Anxanil
- Apo-Hydroxyzine
- Atarax
- Hydrophed
- Marax
- Marax DF
- Multipax
- Novo-Hydroxyzin
- Vistaril

## Uses

- Anxiety Disorder *Guide 106*
- Alcohol withdrawal *Guide 302*
- Relieves tension and agitation
- Relieves symptoms such as itching from allergic reactions

## Dosages

- Tablet
- Syrup
- Capsule

## Overdose Symptoms

- Drowsiness
- Unsteady gait
- Agitation
- Tremors
- Convulsions

## Side Effects/Adverse Reactions

- Nausea
- Dry mouth, nose, throat
- Drowsiness
- Dizziness
- Vision changes
- Incoordination
- Rash
- Painful or difficult urination
- Loss of appetite

## Drug Interactions

*Antidepressants — Tricyclic* Guide 203

- Effects of both drugs increased

*Clozapine* Guide 220

- Toxic effect on the CNS

*Antihistamines* Guide 205

- Hydroxyzine effect increased

*Attapulgite*

- Decreased hydroxyzine effect

*CNS Depressants*

- Greater depression of CNS

## Other Interactions

*Alcohol* Guide 302

- Increased intoxication and sedation

*Caffeine*

- Decreased tranquilizer effect of hydroxyzine

*Cocaine* Guide 307

- Decreased effect of hydroxyzine

---

## (GUIDE 228) LEVODOPA

### Description

- Antiparkinsonism
- Generic available
- Nonaddictive

### Generic & Brand Names

*Generic*

- Levodopa

*Brand*

- Dopar
- Larodopa

### Uses

- Parkinson's Disease *Guide 126*

### Dosages

- Tablet
- Capsule

### Overdose Symptoms

- Muscular twitching
- Spastic eye closure
- Nausea — vomiting
- Diarrhea

- Cardiac arrhythmias
- Tachycardia
- Disorientation
- Hallucinations
- Coma

## Side Effects/Adverse Reactions

- Uncontrollable body movements
- Mood changes
- Diarrhea
- Depression *Guide 113*
- Anxiety *Guide 106*
- Dry mouth

## Drug Interactions

*Antidepressants — Tricyclic Guide 203*

- Possible hypotension

*MAO Inhibitors Guide 231*

- Dangerous hypertension

## Other Interactions

*Cocaine Guide 307*

- Risk of cardiac arrhythmias

## (GUIDE 229) LITHIUM

### Description

- Mood stabilizer
- Generic available
- Nonaddictive
- May correct chemical imbalance in brain's transmission of nerve impulses that deal with mood and behavior

### Generic & Brand Names

*Generic*

- Lithium

*Brand*

- Carbolith
- Cibalith-S
- Duralith
- Eskalith
- Eskalith CR
- Lithane
- Lithizine
- Lithobid
- Lithonate
- Lithotabs

### Uses

- Bipolar Disorder *Guide 107*
- Conduct Disorder *Guide 108*
- Obsessive Compulsive Disorder *Guide 122*
- Schizoid Personality Disorder *Guide 127*
- Alcohol toxicity and addiction *Guide 302*

### Dosages

- Tablet
- Capsule
- Syrup
- Extended-release tablets

## Overdose Symptoms

- Vomiting
- Muscle weakness
- Convulsions
- Stupor
- Coma

## Side Effects/Adverse Reactions

- Dizziness
- Nausea—vomiting
- Diarrhea
- Tremors—shakes
- Dry mouth
- Impotence
- Increased urination
- Anorexia *Guide 116*

## Drug Interactions

*Acetazolamide*

- Decreased lithium effect

*Antihistamines Guide 205*

- Possible excessive sedation

*Bupropion Guide 213*

- Increased risk of seizures

## Other Interactions

*Alcohol Guide 302*

- Possible lithium poisoning

*Cocaine Guide 307*

- Possible psychosis

*Marijuana Guide 318*

- Increased tremor
- Possible psychosis

2

---

# GUIDE 230 LOXAPINE

## Description

- Tranquilizer, antidepressant
- Generic available
- Nonaddictive

## Generic & Brand Names

*Generic*

- Loxapine

*Brand*

- Loxapac
- Loxitane
- Loxitane C

## Uses

- Anxiety Disorder *Guide 106*
- Depression *Guide 113*
- Dissociative Identity Disorder *Guide 114*
- Paranoia *Guide 125*
- Schizophrenia *Guide 131*

## Dosages

- Tablets
- Capsule
- Liquid

## Overdose Symptoms

- Dizziness
- Acute shortness of breath
- Drowsiness
- Muscle spasms
- Coma

## Side Effects/Adverse Reactions

- Serious shortness of breath
- Cardiac arrhythmias
- Excess perspiration
- Skin rash
- Seizure (rare)

## Drug Interactions

*Anticonvulsants*

- Decreases effect of anticonvulsant

*Antidepressants — Tricyclic Guide 203*

- Can increase toxic effects of both medications

*Bupropion Guide 213*

- Increases risk of seizures

*CNS Depressants*

- Increases sedative effects of both medicines

*Epinephrine*

- Tachycardia
- Dangerous hypotension

## Other Interactions

*Alcohol Guide 302*

- Decreases effect of Loxitane

*Cocaine Guide 307*

- Can increase toxicity of both drugs

*Marijuana Guide 318*

- Can increase toxicity of both drugs

*Tobacco*

- Can increase toxicity

# GUIDE 231 MAO INHIBITORS

## Description

- MAO inhibitor
- No generic available
- Nonaddictive
- Inhibits nerve transmissions in brain that may cause depression

## Generic & Brand Names

*Generic*

- Phenelzine
- Tranylcypromine

## Brand

- *Nardil*
- Parnate

## Uses

- Depression *Guide 113*
- Dissociative Identity Disorder *Guide 114*
- Panic Disorder *Guide 124*
- Personality Disorders *Guide 127*
- Migraine headaches

## Dosage

- Tablet

## Overdose Symptoms

- Restlessness
- Irritability
- Agitation
- Fever
- Confusion
- Dizziness
- Cardiac arrhythmias
- Hallucinations
- Difficulty breathing
- Insomnia
- Seizures
- Coma

## Side Effects/Adverse Reactions

- Fatigue/weakness
- Restlessness
- Tremors
- Dry mouth
- Constipation
- Blurred vision

## Drug Interactions

*Amphetamines Guide 202*

- Dangerous hypertension

*Antidepressants — Tricyclic Guide 203*

- Dangerous hypertension
- Possible fever
- Convulsions
- Delirium
- Cardiac arrhythmias

*Antidiabetic Agents — Oral and Insulin*

- Dangerously low blood sugar

*Antihypertensives*

- Dangerous hypotension

*Buspirone Guide 214*

- Hypertension

*Carbamazepine Guide 215*

- Fever
- Seizures

*Citalopram*

- Potential life-threatening reaction

*Clozapine Guide 220*

- Toxic to CNS

*Dextromethorphan Guide 309*

- Potential life-threatening reaction

2

*Diuretics*
- Excessive hypotension

## Other Interactions

*Alcohol* Guide 302
- Increases sedation to dangerous levels

*Amphetamines* Guide 303
- Dangerous hypertension

*Caffeine*
- Cardiac arrhythmias
- Hypertension

*Cocaine* Guide 307
- Extreme stimulation
- Potentially fatal

*Cough Medicine OTC (Over the Counter)* Guide 309
- Potential life-threatening reaction

*Foods Containing Tyramine*
- Excessive hypertension

*Alcoholic Beverages*
- Red wines
- Beer/ale

*Breads*
- Homemade breads high in yeast
- Breads or crackers containing cheese

*Fruits*
- Bananas
- Red plums
- Avocados
- Figs
- Raisins
- Raspberries

*Fats*
- Sour cream

*Marijuana* Guide 318
- Overstimulation

## GUIDE 232 MAPROTILINE

## Description
- Antidepressant
- Generic available
- Nonaddictive

## Generic & Brand Names

*Generic*
- Maprotiline

*Brand*
- Ludiomil

## Uses
- Depression *Guide 113*
- Dissociative Identity Disorder *Guide 114*
- Anxiety associated with depression

## Dosage

- Tablet

## Overdose Symptoms

- Hyperthermia
- Respiratory arrest
- Cardiac arrhythmia
- Muscular stiffness
- Hallucinations
- Seizure
- Coma

## Side Effects/Adverse Reactions

- Seizures
- Tremors
- Headache
- Dry mouth
- Bad taste in mouth
- Constipation
- Diarrhea
- Nausea

## Drug Interactions

*Antiglaucoma Agents*

- Cardiac dysrhythmia
- Hypertension

*Bupropion Guide 213*

- Increases risk of seizures

*CNS Depressants*

- Increases sedation

*Clozapine Guide 220*

- Toxic effect on CNS

*Ethchlorvynol*

- Delirium *Guide 111*

*Narcotics*

- Dangerous level of sedation

## Other Interactions

*Alcohol Guide 302*

- Excessive intoxication

*Cocaine Guide 307*

- Excessive intoxication

*Marijuana Guide 318*

- Excessive drowsiness

---

## (GUIDE 233) MEPROBAMATE

### Description

- Tranquilizer, antianxiety
- Generic available
- Addictive
- Sedates brain centers controlling behavior and emotions

### Generic & Brand Names

*Generic*

- Meprobamate

*Brand*

- Acabamate

- Apo-Meprobamate
- Equanil
- Equanil Wyseals
- Medi-Tran
- Meprospan 200
- Meprospan 400
- Miltown
- Neuramate
- Novomepro
- Novo-Mepro
- Pax 400
- Probate
- Sedabamate
- Trancot
- Tranmep

## Uses

- Mild anxiety reduction
  *Guide 106*
- Dissociative Identity
  Disorder *Guide 114*
- Tension reduction
- Insomnia

## Dosages

- Tablet
- Extended-release capsules

## Overdose Symptoms

- Dizziness
- Slurred speech
- Confusion
- Stumbling gate
- Depressed breathing
- Depressed heart function
- Stupor
- Coma

## Side Effects/Adverse Reactions

- Hives/rash
- Severe itching
- Faintness
- Wheezing—anaphylaxis
- Dizziness
- Agitation
- Drowsiness
- Fatigue/weakness

## Drug Interactions

*Antidepressants—Tricyclic*
*Guide 203*

- Increases antidepressant
  effect

*CNS Depressants*

- Increases depressive effects
  of both medicines

*MAO Inhibitors Guide 231*

- Increases Meprobamate
  effects

## Other Interactions

*Alcohol Guide 302*

- Dangerous increase of
  Meprobamate effect

*Cocaine Guide 307*

- Decreases Meprobamate
  effect

*Marijuana Guide 318*

- Increases sedative effect of
  Meprobamate

# (GUIDE 234) METHYLPHENIDATE

## Description

- CNS stimulant
- Generic available
- Addictive
- Stimulates brain to improve alertness, concentration, and attention span

## Generic & Brand Names

*Generic*

- Methylphenidate
- Dexmethylphenidate

*Brand*

- Concerta
- Focalin
- Metadate CD
- Metadate ER
- Methylin ER
- PMS Methylphenidate
- Ritalin
- Ritalin LA
- Ritalin SR

## Uses

- ADD/ADHD *Guide 103*
- Adult Depression *Guide 113*
- Narcolepsy *Guide 121*

## Dosages

- Tablet
- Extended-release tablet
- Extended-release capsule

## Overdose Symptoms

- Tachycardia
- Fever
- Confusion
- Vomiting
- Agitation
- Hallucinations
- Seizures
- Coma

## Side Effects/Adverse Reactions

- Nervousness
- Difficulty sleeping
- Dizziness
- Nausea
- Headache
- Abdominal pain
- Weight loss
- Drowsiness
- Agitated delirium

## Psychotropic & Other Medication Interactions

*Anticholinergics*

- Increased anticholinergic effect

*Anticoagulants — Oral*

- Increased anticoagulant effect

*Anticonvulsants*

- Increased anticonvulsant effect
- Decreased stimulant effect

### Antidepressants — Tricyclic
*Guide 203*

- Increased antidepressant effect
- Decreased stimulant effect

### Antihypertensives

- Decreased antihypertensive effect

### CNS stimulants

- Overstimulation

### Dextrothyroxine

- Increased stimulation

### MAO Inhibitors *Guide 231*

- Dangerous hypertension

## Other Interactions

### Caffeine

- Hypertension

### Cocaine *Guide 307*

- Cardiac arrhythmias
- Hypertension

---

## GUIDE 235 · MIRTAZAPINE

### Description

- Antidepressant
- No generic available
- Nonaddictive

### Generic & Brand Names

#### Generic

- None

#### Brand

- Remeron
- Remeron SolTab

### Uses

- Depression *Guide 113*
- Dissociative Identity Disorder *Guide 114*

### Dosage

- Tablet

### Overdose Symptoms

- Drowsiness
- Disorientation
- Impaired memory
- Tachycardia

### Side Effects/Adverse Reactions

- Sleepiness
- Increased appetite
- Weight gain
- Constipation
- Sexual side effects

## Drug Interactions

*MAO Inhibitors* Guide 231

* Potential life-threatening reaction

*Benzodiazepines* Guide 210

* Increased sedation

## Other Interactions

*Alcohol* Guide 302

* Increases sedation

**2**

## GUIDE 236 MODAFINIL (PROVIGIL)

### Description

* Antinarcoleptic, CNS stimulant
* No generic available
* Addictive

### Generic & Brand Names

*Generic*

* Modafinil

*Brand*

* Provigil

### Use

* Narcolepsy *Guide 121*

### Dosage

* Tablet

### Overdose Symptoms

* Usually non-life-threatening

* Agitation
* Hypertension
* Tachycardia
* Insomnia

### Side Effects/Adverse Reactions

* Anxiety
* Headache
* Nausea
* Insomnia

### Drug Interactions

*Antidepressants*

* Increased effects

*CNS Stimulants*

* Increased effects of stimulant

## (GUIDE 237) MOLINDONE

### Description
- Antipsychotic
- No generic available
- Nonaddictive
- Treats imbalance in nerve impulses from the brain

### Generic & Brand Names

*Generic*
- Molindone

*Brand*
- Moban
- Moban Concentrate

### Uses
- Severe anxiety *Guide 106*
- Conduct Disorder *Guide 108*
- Paranoia *Guide 125*
- Schizophrenia *Guide 131*

### Dosages
- Tablet
- Liquid

### Overdose Symptoms
- Stupor
- Seizures
- Coma

### Side Effects/Adverse Reactions
- High fever
- Tachycardia
- Excessive perspiration
- Muscular rigidity
- Seizures
- Confusion
- Irritability

### Drug Interactions

*Bupropion Guide 213*
- Increases risk of seizures

*Clozapine Guide 220*
- Toxic effects on CNS

*Fluoxetine Guide 249*
- Increases depression

*Loxapine Guide 230*
- Can increase toxic effects of both drugs

### Other Interactions

*Alcohol Guide 302*
- Oversedation

*Marijuana Guide 318*
- Increased drowsiness

## Description

- Antidepressant
- No generic available
- Nonaddictive
- Appears to block reuptake of serotonin and norepinephrine in the brain

## Generic & Brand Names

### Generic

- Nefazodone

### Brand

- Serzone

## Uses

- Depression  *Guide 113*
- Dissociative Identity Disorder *Guide 114*

## Dosage

- Tablet

## Overdose Symptoms

- Drowsiness
- Nausea—vomiting
- Hypotension

## Side Effects/Adverse Reactions

- Incoordination
- Blurred vision
- Fainting
- Ringing in ears
- Strange dreams
- Constipation
- Diarrhea
- Skin rash

## Drug Interactions

### Antihypertensives

- Potential serious hypotension

### Astemizole

- Cardiac arrhythmias
- Serious heart problems

### MAO Inhibitors *Guide 231*

- Possibly life-threatening

### Selective Serotonin Reuptake Inhibitors (SSRIs) *Guide 249*

- Potential life-threatening serotonin syndrome

### Terfenadine

- Cardiac arrhythmias
- Serious heart problems

## Other Interactions

### Alcohol *Guide 302*

- Oversedation

## Description

- Binds to opioid receptors in the CNS and blocks the effects of narcotic drugs
- Generic available
- Nonaddictive

## Generic & Brand Names

*Generic*

- Naltrexone

*Brand*

- Barr
- ReVia

## Uses

- Treatment of detoxified narcotics addicts—helps to maintain a drug-free state
- Alcoholism (in conjunction with counseling) *Guide 302*

## Dosage

- Tablets

## Overdose Symptoms

- Seizure
- Coma

## Side Effects/Adverse Reactions

- Hallucinations
- Tachycardia
- Fainting
- Difficulty breathing
- Insomnia
- Anxiety
- Headache
- Nausea
- Vomiting
- Skin rash
- Chills
- Constipation

## Drug Interactions

*Narcotic Medicines*

- Precipitates withdrawal symptoms
- Possible cardiac arrest
- Coma
- Death (if Naltrexone is taken while patient is dependent on this class of drugs)

*Isoniazid*

- Increased risk of liver damage

## Other Interactions

*Alcohol Guide 302*

- Unpredictable effects

*Cocaine Guide 307*

- Unpredictable effects

*Marijuana Guide 318*

- Unpredictable effects

# (GUIDE 240) NIACIN

## Description

- Vitamin B-3: nicotinic acid
- Vasodilator, antihyperlipidemic
- Generic available
- Nonaddictive

## Generic & Brand Names

- Advicor
- Endur-Acin
- Nia-Bid
- Niac
- Niacels
- Niacin
- Niacor
- Nico-400
- Nicobid
- Nicolar
- Nicotinex
- Nicotinyl
- Papulex
- Roniacol
- Ronigen
- Rycotin
- Slo-Niacin
- Span-Niacin
- Tega-Span
- Tri-B3

## Uses

- Parkinson's Disease
  Guide 126
- Niacin replacement
- Vertigo
- Prevention of premenstrual headaches
- Cholesterol reduction
- Triglyceride reduction
- Pellagra

## Dosages

- Tablet
- Liquid

## Overdose Symptoms

- Flushed features
- Nausea—vomiting
- Stomach cramps
- Light-headedness
- Fainting
- Sweating

## Side Effects/Adverse Reactions

- Dry skin
- Upper abdominal pain
- Diarrhea
- Allergic reaction

## Drug Interactions

*Beta-Blockers* Guide 211

- Dangerous hypotension

*Mecamylamine*

- Dangerous hypotension

*Methyldopa*

- Dangerous hypotension

## Other Interactions

*Alcohol* Guide 302

- Dangerous hypotension

## (GUIDE 241) OLANZAPINE

### Description

- Antipsychotic
- No generic available
- Nonaddictive
- Blocks certain nerve impulses

### Generic & Brand Names

*Generic*

- Olanzapine

*Brand*

- Zyprexa

### Uses

- Acute mania *Guide 107*
- Conduct Disorder *Guide 108*
- Paranoia *Guide 125*
- Schizophrenia *Guide 131*
- Tourette's Disorder *Guide 136*

### Dosage

- Tablet

### Overdose Symptoms

- Slurred speech
- Drowsiness

### Side Effects/Adverse Reactions

- High fever
- Tachycardia
- Excessive perspiration
- Muscular rigidity
- Seizures—rare

### Drug Interactions

*Hepatoxins*

- Increased risk of liver problems

### Other Interactions

*Alcohol Guide 302*

- Increases sedation

## (GUIDE 242) ORPHENADRINE

### Description

- Muscle relaxant, antiparkinsonism
- Generic available
- Possibly addictive

### Generic & Brand Names

*Generic*

- Orphenadrine

*Brand*

- Banflex
- Blanex
- Disipal
- Flexagin
- Flexoject
- Flexon
- K-Flex
- Marflex
- Myolin

- Myotrol
- Neocyten
- Noradex
- O-Flex
- Orflagen
- Orfro
- Orphenate
- Tega-Flex

## Uses

- Muscle strains
- Parkinson's Disease
  *Guide 126*

## Dosages

- Tablet
- Extended-release tablet

## Overdose Symptoms

- Fainting
- Disorientation
- Difficulty breathing
- Dilated pupils
- Tachycardia
- Paralysis
- Seizures
- Coma

## Side Effects/Adverse Reactions

- Transient paralysis
- Severe weakness
- Temporary loss of vision
- Hives, rash, severe itching

## Drug Interactions

### *Chlorpromazine*

- Low blood sugar

### *Nabilone*

- Increased depression
  *Guide 113*

### *Propoxyphene*

- Confusion, nervousness, tremors

## Other Interactions

### *Alcohol* *Guide 302*

- Increased drowsiness

### *Marijuana* *Guide 318*

- Increased drowsiness
- Dry mouth
- Fainting
- Muscular weakness

# (GUIDE 243) PEMOLINE

## Description

- CNS stimulant
- No generic available
- Addictive
- Decreases overactivity and lengthens attention span

## Generic & Brand Names

### *Generic*

- Pemoline

### *Brand*

- Cylert

## Uses
* ADHD *Guide 103*

## Dosages
* Tablet
* Chewable tablet

## Overdose Symptoms
* Agitation
* Confusion
* Tachycardia
* Hallucinations
* Severe headache
* High fever
* Dilated pupils
* Muscle twitching/trembling
* Uncontrolled eye or body movements

## Side Effects/Adverse Reactions
* Insomnia
* Loss of appetite

* Weight loss
* Irritability
* Depression

## Drug Interactions
### Anticonvulsants
* Increased likelihood of depression

### CNS Stimulants
* May increase toxic effect of both drugs

## Other Interactions
### Alcohol *Guide 302*
* Increases chance of depression

### Caffeine
* Overstimulation

---

# GUIDE 244  PERGOLIDE

## Description
* Antidyskinetic
* No generic available
* Nonaddictive
* Stimulates dopamine receptors

## Generic & Brand Names
### Generic
* Pergolide

### Brand
* Permax

## Uses
### Parkinson's Disease
*Guide 126*

* In conjunction with Levodopa *Guide 228*
* In conjunction with Carbidopa and Levodopa *Guide 216*

## Dosage

- Tablet

## Overdose Symptoms

- None expected
- If present, non-life-threatening

## Side Effects/Adverse Reactions

- Angina
- Seizures
- Shortness of breath
- Disorientation
- Hallucinations
- Unusual motor activity

## Drug Interactions

*Hypotension-causing Drugs*

- Increases hypotensive effects

*Sertraline Guide 249*

- Can increase depressive effects of both

## Other Interactions

*Alcohol Guide 302*

- Increased chance of adverse reactions

*Cocaine Guide 307*

- Increased chance of adverse reactions

*Marijuana Guide 318*

- Increased chance of adverse reactions

2

---

## GUIDE 245 — PHENOTHIAZINES

### Description

- Tranquilizer, antiemetic
- Generic available
- Nonaddictive
- Suppresses abnormal emotions and behavior brain centers

### Generic & Brand Names

*Generic*

- Acetophenazine
- Chlorpromazine
- Fluphenazine
- Mesoridazine
- Methotrimeprazine
- Pericyazine
- Perphenazine
- Pipotiazine
- Prochlorperazine
- Promazine
- Thiopropazate
- Thioproperazine
- Thioridazine
- Trifluoperazine
- Triflupromazine

### *Brand*

- Apo-Fluphenazine
- Apo-Perphenazine
- Apo-Thioridazine
- Apo-Trifluoperazine
- Chlorpromanyl-5
- Chlorpromanyl-20
- Chlorpromanyl-40
- Compazine
- Compazine Spansule
- Dartal
- Duo-Medihaler
- Elavil Plus
- Etrafon
- Etrafon-A
- Etrafon-D
- Etrafon-F
- Etrafon-Forte
- Largactil
- Largactil Liquid
- Largactil Oral Drops
- Levoprome
- Majeptil
- Mellaril
- Mellaril Concentrate
- Mellaril-S
- Modecate
- Modecate Concentrate
- Moditen Enanthate
- Moditen HCI
- Moditen HCI-H.P.
- Neuleptil
- Novo-Chlorpromazine
- Novo-Flurazine
- Novo-Ridazine
- Nozinan
- Nozinan Liquid
- Nozinan Oral Drops
- Permitil
- Permitil Concentrate
- Piportil L4
- PMS Levazine
- PMS Thioridazine
- Prolixin
- Prolixin Concentrate
- Prolixin Decanoate
- Prolixin Enanthate
- Prorazin
- Prozine
- Serentil
- Serentil Concentrate
- Solazine
- Stelazine
- Stelazine Concentrate
- Stemetil
- Stemetil Liquid
- Suprazine
- Terfluzine
- Terfluzine Concentrate
- Thorazine
- Thorazine Concentrate
- Thorazine Spansule
- Thor-Prom
- Tindal
- Triavil
- Trilafon
- Trilafon Concentrate
- Ultrazine-10
- Vesprin

## Uses

- Anxiety Disorder *Guide 106*
- Paranoia *Guide 125*
- Schizophrenia *Guide 131*
- Agitation
- Stops nausea, vomiting, and hiccups

## Dosages

- Tablets
- Drops/liquid
- Suppositories

## Overdose Symptoms

- Stupor
- Seizures
- Coma

## Side Effects/Adverse Reactions

- High fever
- Tachycardia
- Excessive perspiration
- Irritability
- Confusion
- Seizures
- Dry mouth
- Dizziness

- Hypotension
- Movement disorders

## Drug Interactions

*Anticonvulsants*

- Increased risk of seizures

*Antihypertensives*

- Severe hypotension

*Bupropion* Guide 213

- Increased risk of seizures

## Other Interactions

*Alcohol* Guide 302

- Dangerous oversedation

*Marijuana* Guide 318

- Drowsiness
- Can increase antinausea effect

## GUIDE 246 QUETIAPINE (SEROQUEL)

## Description

- Antipsychotic
- No generic available
- Nonaddictive

## Generic & Brand Names

*Generic*

- Quetiapine

*Brand*

- Seroquel

## Uses

- Conduct Disorder *Guide 108*

- Paranoia *Guide 125*
- Schizophrenia *Guide 131*

## Dosage

- Tablet

## Overdose Symptoms

- Slurred speech
- Drowsiness

## Side Effects/Adverse Reactions

- High fever
- Tachycardia
- Excessive perspiration
- Muscular rigidity
- Movement disorders

- Disorientation
- Seizures

## Drug Interactions

*CNS Depressants*

- May increase sedation

## Other Interactions

*Alcohol Guide 302*

- May increase sedation

---

## (GUIDE 247) RISPERIDONE

### Description

- Antipsychotic
- No generic available
- Nonaddictive
- May block certain nerve impulses between nerve cells

### Generic & Brand Names

*Generic*

- Risperidone

*Brand*

- Risperdal

### Uses

- Conduct Disorder *Guide 108*
- Paranoia *Guide 125*
- Schizophrenia *Guide 131*
- Tourette's Disorder *Guide 136*
- Bipolar Disorder *Guide 107*

### Dosages

- Tablet
- Oral solution

### Overdose Symptoms

- Extreme drowsiness
- Tachycardia
- Faintness
- Seizures
- Profuse perspiration
- Difficulty breathing
- Loss of muscular coordination

### Side Effects/Adverse Reactions

- High fever
- Tachycardia
- Profuse sweating
- Muscle rigidity
- Confusion and irritability
- Seizures
- Anxiety
- Dizziness
- Digestive problems
- Rash
- Sexual dysfunction

### Drug Interactions

*Antihypertensives*

- Increased antihypertensive effect

### Other Interactions

*Alcohol Guide 302*

- Increased sedation

## Description

- Antidyskinetic
- Generic available
- Nonaddictive
- Inhibits action of monoamine oxidase type B (MAO B)

## Generic & Brand Names

*Generic*

- Selegiline

*Brand*

- Carbex
- Eldepryl
- Jumax
- Jumexal
- Juprenil
- Movergan
- Procythol
- SD Deprenyl

## Uses

- Depression *Guide 113*

*Parkinson's Disease*
*Guide 126*

- In conjunction with Levodopa *Guide 228*
- In conjunction with Carbidopa and Levodopa *Guide 216*

## Dosages

- Tablets

## Overdose Symptoms

- Difficulty opening mouth
- Muscle spasm
- Sweating
- Irregular tachycardia
- Hyperactive reflexes
- Chest pain
- Fainting
- Seizures
- Coma

## Side Effects/Adverse Reactions

- Chest pain
- Dilated pupils
- Cardiac arrhythmia
- Neck pain
- Nausea—vomiting
- Mood changes

## Drug Interactions

*Meperidine*

- Potential severe hypotension

*Narcotics*

- Toxic reactions
- Seizures
- Coma
- Death

## Other Interactions

*Alcohol Guide 302*

- Severe toxicity

*Cocaine* Guide 307

- Hypertension
- Tachycardia

*Foods Containing Tyramine*

- Severe toxicity
- Possibly fatal

*Beverages*

- Alcoholic beverages
- Red wines
- Beer/ale

*Breads*

- Homemade breads high in yeast
- Breads or crackers containing cheese

*Fruits*

- Bananas
- Red plums
- Avocados
- Figs
- Raisins
- Raspberries

*Fats*

- Sour cream

*Marijuana* Guide 318

- Tachycardia

*Tobacco*

- Tachycardia

---

## GUIDE 249 — SELECTIVE SEROTONIN REUPTAKE INHIBITORS (SSRIs)

### Description

- Antidepressant, antiobsessional, and antianxiety agent
- Some generics available
- Nonaddictive
- Selective serotonin reuptake inhibitors—enhance serotonin level in the brain

### Generic & Brand Names

*Generic*

- Citalopram
- Escitalopram
- Fluoxetine
- Fluvoxamine
- Paroxetine
- Sertraline

*Brand*

- Celexa
- Lexapro
- Prozac
- Prozac Weekly
- Sarafem
- Paxil
- Paxil CR
- Zoloft

### Uses

- Paroxetine used for anxiety *Guide 106*
- Depression *Guide 113*

- Dissociative Identity Disorder *Guide 114*
- Fluoxetine and Fluoxamine used for Bulimia *Guide 116*
- Obsessive Compulsive Disorder *Guide 122*
- Personality Disorders *Guide 127*
- Phobias *Guide 129*
- Paroxetine used for PTSD *Guide 130*
- Separation Anxiety Disorder *Guide 132*
- Tourette's Disorder *Guide 136*
- Premenstrual Dysphoric Disorder

## Dosages

- Capsules
- Tablets
- Liquid

## Overdose Symptoms

- Dizziness
- Excessive perspiration
- Nausea—vomiting
- Tremors
- Cardiac arrhythmias
- Amnesia—rare
- Coma—rare
- Seizures—rare

## Side Effects/Adverse Reactions

- Rash
- Itchy skin
- Difficulty breathing
- Chest pain
- Drowsiness
- Nausea
- Coughing
- Lower back and side pain
- Insomnia

## Drug Interactions

*Anticoagulants—Oral*

- Increases risk of side effects for both medications

*Antidepressants—Tricyclic Guide 203*

- Increases risk of side effects for both medications

*MAO Inhibitors Guide 231*

- Hypotensive/hypertensive crisis
- Increases risk of side effects
- Seizures

## Other Interactions

*Alcohol Guide 302*

- Contributes to depression *Guide 113*

---

## GUIDE 250 THIAMINE (VITAMIN B-1)

### Description

- Vitamin supplement
- Generic available
- Nonaddictive
- Promotes normal growth and development

- Combines with an enzyme to metabolize carbohydrates

## Generic & Brand Names

*Generic*

- Thiamine (Vitamin B-1)

*Brand*

- Betalin S
- Betaxin
- Bewon
- Biamine

## Uses

- Alcoholism *Guide 302*
- Absorption Diseases
- Beri-Beri—thiamine deficiency disease
- Breast-feeding
- Burns
- Cirrhosis
- Dietary supplement
- Hyperthyroidism
- Infection
- Pregnancy
- Prolonged diarrhea

## Dosages

- Tablet
- Liquid

## Overdose Symptoms

- Unlikely to threaten life

## Side Effects/Adverse Reactions

- Hives
- Rash
- Intense itching
- Faintness
- Wheezing
- Allergic reaction

## Drug Interactions

*Barbiturates Guide 209*

- Decreased thiamine effect

## Other Interactions

*Beverages: Carbonates & Citrates*

- Decreased thiamine effect

*Foods: Carbonates & Citrates*

- Decreased thiamine effect

# GUIDE 251 · THIOTHIXENE

## Description

- Antipsychotic
- Generic available
- Nonaddictive
- Correction of nerve impulses

## Generic & Brand Names

*Generic*

- Thiothixene

## Brand

- Navane
- Thiothixene HCI Intensol

## Uses

- Severe anxiety *Guide 106*
- Paranoia *Guide 125*
- Schizophrenia *Guide 131*
- Agitation

## Dosages

- Capsule
- Syrup

## Overdose Symptoms

- Confusion
- Blurred vision
- Tachycardia
- Shallow breathing
- Hypotension
- Convulsions
- Coma

## Side Effects/Adverse Reactions

- High fever
- Tachycardia
- Excess perspiration
- Muscle rigidity
- Confusion
- Irritability
- Seizures
- Spastic movements
- Pacing/restlessness

- Difficulty urinating
- Blurred vision

## Drug Interactions

### Anticonvulsants

- Seizure pattern changes

### Antidepressants — Tricyclic
*Guide 203*

- Excessive sedation
- Increases effects of thiothixene

### Antihistamines *Guide 205*

- Extreme hypotension

### Bupropion *Guide 213*

- Increases chances of seizures

### Epinephrine

- Extreme hypotension

### MAO Inhibitors *Guide 231*

- Excessive sedation

## Other Interactions

- Alcohol *Guide 302*
- Excessive brain depression

### Marijuana *Guide 308*

- Daily use—fainting and possible psychosis

## GUIDE 252  TOLCAPONE

### Description

- Antidyskinetic, anti-parkinsonism
- No generic available
- Nonaddictive
- Increases blood levels of Levodopa and Carbidopa for necessary normal nerve impulses

### Generic & Brand Names

*Generic*

- Tolcapone

*Brand*

- Tasmar

### Uses

*Parkinson's Disease Guide 126*

- In conjunction with Levodopa *Guide 228*
- In conjunction with Carbidopa and Levodopa *Guide 216*

### Dosage

- Tablet

### Overdose Symptoms

- Nausea—vomiting
- Dizziness

### Side Effects/Adverse Reactions

- Stomach pain
- Decreased appetite
- Diarrhea
- Twitching
- Fainting
- Nausea—vomiting
- Constipation

### Drug Interactions

*Desipramine Guide 203*

- May increase adverse effects of Tolcapone

### Other Interactions

*Alcohol Guide 302*

- Possible hallucinations

*Cocaine Guide 307*

- Possible hallucinations

*Marijuana Guide 318*

- Possible hallucinations

## GUIDE 253  TRAZODONE

### Description

- Antidepressant (nontricyclic); inhibits serotonin uptake in the brain
- Generic available
- Nonaddictive

## Generic & Brand Names

### Generic

- Trazodone

### Brand

- Desyrel
- Trazon
- Trialodine

## Uses

- Anxiety disorder *Guide 106*
- Depression *Guide 113*
- Dissociative Identity Disorder *Guide 114*
- Sleep enhancement
- Some types of chronic pain

## Dosage

- Tablet

## Overdose Symptoms

- Respiratory arrest
- Fainting
- Cardiac arrhythmias
- Angina
- Seizures
- Coma

## Side Effects/Adverse Reactions

- Drowsiness

## Drug Interactions

### Antihypertensives

- Dangerous hypotension

### Barbiturates *Guide 209*

- Dangerous hypotension

### Bupropion *Guide 213*

- Increases risk of seizures

## Other Interactions

### Alcohol *Guide 302*

- Oversedation

### Caffeine

- Cardiac arrhythmias

### Marijuana *Guide 318*

- Cardiac arrhythmias

### Tobacco

- Cardiac arrhythmias

2

---

**GUIDE 254** VALPROIC ACID

## Description

- Anticonvulsant
- Generic available
- Nonaddictive
- Increases gamma amino-butyric acid—inhibits nerve transmission in parts of the brain

## Generic & Brand Names

### Generic

- Valproic Acid

### Brand

- Depakene
- Myproic acid

## Uses

- Epilepsy
- Bipolar Disorder—treats the manic phase *Guide 107*
- Conduct Disorder *Guide 108*
- Borderline Personality Disorder *Guide 127*
- Traumatic Brain Injury *Guide 137*

## Dosages

- Capsule
- Syrup

## Overdose Symptoms

- Coma

## Side Effects/Adverse Reactions

- Loss of appetite
- Indigestion
- Nausea or vomiting
- Poor coordination
- Diarrhea
- Weight gain/loss
- Menstrual changes

## Drug Interactions

### Anticoagulants

- Increases risk of bleeding

### Antiinflammatory

- Increases risk of bleeding

### Antivirals—Influenza *Guide 206*

- Increases risk of Pancreatitis

### CNS Depressants

- Increases sedation

### Clonazepam *Guide 210*

- May prolong seizures

## Other Interactions

### Alcohol *Guide 302*

- Deep sedation

### Cocaine *Guide 307*

- Increases brain sensitivity

### Marijuana *Guide 318*

- Increases brain sensitivity

# ( GUIDE 255 ) VENLAFAXINE (EFFEXOR)

## Description

- Antidepressant—Bicyclic
- No Generic available
- Addictive (not known)

## Generic & Brand Names

### Generic

- Venlafaxine

### Brand

- Effexor
- Effexor XR

## Uses

- Anxiety Disorders *Guide 106*
- Depression *Guide 113*
- Dissociative Identity Disorder *Guide 114*
- Phobias *Guide 129*
- PTSD *Guide 130*

## Dosages

- Tablet
- Extended release capsule

## Overdose Symptoms

- Possibly no symptoms
- Extreme drowsiness
- Convulsions
- Tachycardia

## Side Effects/Adverse Reactions

- Tachycardia
- Blurred vision
- Hypertension
- Stomach pain
- Intestinal gas
- Insomnia
- Drowsiness
- Decreased sex drive
- Impotence
- Nausea—vomiting
- Constipation
- Dry mouth
- Fatigue
- Sweating
- Nervousness
- Tremors
- Headache

## Drug Interactions

### Antidepressants

- Increases sedative effect

### CNS Depressants

- Increases sedative effect

### MAO Inhibitors *Guide 231*

- Increases risk and severity of adverse reactions

## Other Interactions

### Alcohol *Guide 302*

- Increases sedative effect

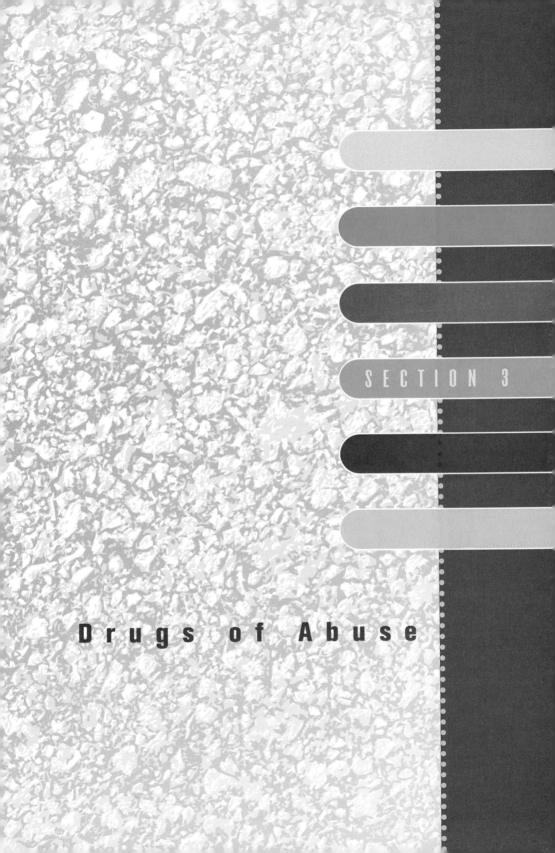

SECTION 3

Drugs of Abuse

3

| | | |
|---|---|---|
| Arcet | 304 | **170** |
| Arnolds | 328 | **216** |
| Astromorph | 320 | **200** |
| Astromorph-PF | 320 | **200** |
| Ativan | 305 | **173** |
| Avinza | 320 | **200** |
| Axotal | 304 | **170** |
| Azma Aid | 304 | **170** |
| Bagging | 315 | **194** |
| Bancap | 304 | **170** |
| Barbita | 304 | **170** |
| Barbiturates | 304 | **170** |
| Barbs | 304 | **171** |
| Bayhistine DH | 308 | **179** |
| Bayhistine Expectorant | 308 | **179** |
| Baytussin AC | 308 | **179** |
| Baytussin Expectorant | 308 | **179** |
| Benylin with Codeine | 308 | **179** |
| Benzodiazepines | 305 | **173** |
| Blow | 307 | **177** |
| Blunt | 318 | **196** |
| Boat | 324 | **209** |
| Boom | 313 | **189** |
| Boomers | 321 | **203** |
| Bromanyl | 308 | **179** |
| Bromazepam | 305 | **172** |
| Bronkolixir | 304 | **170** |
| Bronkotabs | 304 | **170** |
| Brontex | 308 | **179** |
| Brown Sugar | 314 | **191** |
| Bucet | 304 | **170** |
| Bump | 307 | **177** |
| Busodium | 304 | **170** |

3

3

3

3

3

| | | |
|---|---:|---:|
| Moon Gas | 315 | 194 |
| Morph | 320 | 200 |
| Morphine | 320 | 200 |
| Morphitec | 320 | 200 |
| MS Contin | 320 | 200 |
| MSIR | 320 | 200 |
| MST Continus | 320 | 200 |
| Mudrane GG | 304 | 171 |
| Murder 8 | 311 | 185 |
| Mushrooms | 321 | 203 |
| Mytussin AC | 308 | 179 |
| Mytussin DAC | 308 | 179 |
| Narcotic Analgesics | 322 | 204 |
| Nembutal | 304 | 171 |
| Neo-Pause | 328 | 216 |
| Nitrazepam | 305 | 172 |
| Nitrites | 315 | 193 |
| Nitrous | 315 | 194 |
| Nitrous Oxide | 315 | 193 |
| Nondrolone | 328 | 215 |
| Nortussin with Codeine | 308 | 179 |
| Notec | 306 | 175 |
| Nova-Rectal | 304 | 171 |
| Novagest Expectorant with Codeine | 308 | 179 |
| Novahistex C | 308 | 179 |
| Novahistine DH Expectorant | 308 | 179 |
| Novahistine DH Liquid | 308 | 179 |
| Novahistine Expectorant | 308 | 179 |
| Novo-Alprazol | 305 | 173 |
| Novochlorhydrate | 306 | 175 |
| Novoclopate | 305 | 173 |
| Novodipam | 305 | 173 |
| Novoflupam | 305 | 173 |

3

3

3

3

## (GUIDE 302) ALCOHOL

### Description

- Clinically significant maladaptive behavior and/or psychological changes related to alcohol use/abuse
- Addictive

### Duration of Effect

- Depends on amount consumed
- The liver can metabolize only about one drink per hour

## Signs & Symptoms

### Intoxication

- Slurred speech
- Loss of coordination
- Unsteady gait
- Nystagmus; unusual eye movement
- Impaired judgment
- Difficulty focusing attention
- Memory impairment
- Irritable to violent
- Distorted vision and/or hearing
- Stupor or coma
- Altered perceptions and emotions
- Hangover

### Overdose

- Loss of consciousness
- Coma
- Respiratory arrest

### Withdrawal

- Tachycardia
- Excessive perspiration
- Hand tremor
- Insomnia
- Nausea or vomiting
- Transient visual, tactile, or auditory hallucinations
- Psychomotor agitation

- Anxiety
- Seizures

## Medications Used in Treatment

### Benzodiazepines *Guide 210*

- Tranquilizer
- Generic available
- Addictive

### Beta-Blockers *Guide 211*

- Antiadrogenic, anti-anginal, antiarrhythmic, antihypertensive
- Generic available
- Nonaddictive

### Buspirone *Guide 214*

- Antianxiety agent
- Generic available
- Nonaddictive

### Carbamazepine (Tegretol) *Guide 215*

- Analgesic, anticonvulsant, antimanic
- Generic available
- Nonaddictive

### Disulfiram (Antabuse) *Guide 221*

- No drug class
- Generic available
- Nonaddictive

### Hydroxyzine *Guide 227*

- Tranquilizer, antihistamine
- Generic available
- Nonaddictive

3

**Lithium** *Guide 229*

- Mood stabilizer
- Generic available
- Nonaddictive

**Naltrexone** *Guide 239*

- Narcotic antagonist
- Generic available
- Nonaddictive

**Thiamine (Vitamin B-1)**
*Guide 250*

- Vitamin supplement
- Generic available
- Nonaddictive

## Psychotropic & Other Medication Reactions

**Amphetamines** *Guide 202*

- Decreased amphetamine effect

**Antidepressants — Tricyclic**
*Guide 203*

- Excessive intoxication

**Antidyskinetics** *Guide 204*

- Excessive sedation

**Antihistamines** *Guide 205*

- Increased sedation

**Antivirals — Influenza** *Guide 206*

- Increased effects of alcohol

**Aripiprazole (Abilify)**
*Guide 207*

- Increased sedation

**Barbiturates** *Guide 209*

- Potentially fatal oversedation

**Bromocriptine** *Guide 212*

- Decreased alcohol tolerance

**Buspirone (BuSpar)**
*Guide 214*

- Excessive sedation

**Clozapine** *Guide 220*

- Toxic to central nervous system (CNS)

**Ergoloid Mesylates** *Guide 223*

- May decrease blood pressure

**Ergotamine, Belladonna, & Phenobarbital** *Guide 224*

- Potentially fatal oversedation

**Haloperidol** *Guide 226*

- Deep sedation and decreased brain function

**Monoamine Oxidase (MAO) Inhibitors** *Guide 231*

- Increased sedation to dangerous levels

**Maprotiline** *Guide 232*

- Excessive intoxication

**Meprobamate** *Guide 233*

- Dangerously increased effect of Meprobamate

3

*Mirtazapine (Remeron)*
Guide 235

• Increased sedation

*Moban* Guide 237

• Increased sedation

*Nefazodone (Serzone)*
Guide 238

• Increased sedation

*Niacin (Vitamin B-3)*
Guide 240

• Dangerous hypotension

*Olanzapine (Zyprexa)*
Guide 241

• Increased sedation

*Orphenadrine* Guide 242

• Increased drowsiness

*Phenothiazines* Guide 245

• Dangerous oversedation

*Selegiline* Guide 248

• Severe toxicity

*Thiothixene* Guide 251

• Excessive brain depression

*Tolcapone* Guide 252

• Possible hallucinations

*Trazodone* Guide 253

• Increased sedation

*Valproic Acid* Guide 254

• Deep sedation

*Venlafaxine (Effexor)*
Guide 255

• Increased sedation

## Other Interactions

*Narcotic Drugs* Guide 322

• Increased intoxicating
  effect of alcohol

## Assessment

• Assess scene safety
  Guide 402
• Use personal protective
  equipment (PPE) Guide 002
• Approach patient Guide 003
• Primary and secondary
  medical survey Guide 403
• Medications
• Brief mental status exam
  Guide 404
• Lethality assessment
  Guide 407
• Emotional first aid
  Guide 004

## Reporting

• Patient description
• Chief complaint
• Medical findings
• Mental status
• Lethality

## Description

- CNS stimulant
- Generic available
- Addictive
- White, odorless, bitter-tasting powder
- May be refined into crystalline "rocks"
- Prescription forms available as tablets or capsules
- Snorted, ingested, injected

### Duration of Effect

- Varies, depending on how administered

## Medical Uses *Guide 202*

- Attention Deficit Hyperactivity Disorder *Guide 103*
- Depression—elderly *Guide 113*
- Narcolepsy *Guide 121*
- Short-term treatment for obesity

## Generic & Brand Names

### Generic

- Amphetamine
- Dextroamphetamine
- Methamphetamine

### Brand

- Adderall
- Adderall XR
- Desoxyn
- Desoxyn Gradumet
- Dexedrine
- Dexedrine Spansule
- Oxydess
- Spancap

## Street Names

- Chalk
- Crank
- Crystal
- Glass
- Ice
- Go Fast
- Meth
- Shit
- Speed
- TSS
- Tweak

## Signs & Symptoms

### Intoxication

- Tachycardia
- Dilated pupils
- Elevated blood pressure
- Perspiration or chills
- Psychomotor agitation
- Muscular tension
- Euphoria
- Hypervigilance
- Paranoia *Guide 125*

### Overdose

- Tachycardia
- Lowered blood pressure
- Lowered respiration
- Chest pain
- Cardiac arrythmias
- Dystonia; muscular weakness

- Confusion
- Dyskinesia; deficits in voluntary movement
- Seizures
- Coma
- Agitated delirium
- Malignant hyperthermia

## Withdrawal

- Depression *Guide 113*
- Fatigue
- Vivid, unpleasant dreams
- Insomnia or hypersomnia
- Increased appetite
- Psychomotor retardation

## Psychotropic & Other Medication Reactions

### Antidepressants — Tricyclic
*Guide 203*

- Decreased amphetamine effect

### Antihypertensives

- Decreased antihypertensive effect

### Beta-Blockers *Guide 211*

- Hypertension, bradycardia

### Carbonic Anhydrase Inhibitors

- Increased amphetamine effect

### CNS Stimulants

- Excessive CNS stimulation

### Furazolidone

- Sudden and severe hypertension

### Sympathomimetics

- Seizures

### Thyroid Hormones

- Cardiac arrhythmias

## Assessment

- Assess scene safety *Guide 402*
- Use PPE *Guide 002*
- Approach patient *Guide 003*
- Primary and secondary medical survey *Guide 403*
- Medications
- Brief mental status exam *Guide 404*
- Lethality assessment *Guide 407*
- Emotional first aid *Guide 004*

## Reporting

- Patient description
- Chief complaint
- Medical findings
- Mental status
- Lethality

3

## Description

- Antiseizure
- Generic available
- Addictive

## Medical Uses *Guide 209*

- Anxiety disorders *Guide 106*
- Epilepsy
- Prevention of febrile seizures
- Sleep aid, short-term basis
- Asthma
- Gastrointestinal disorders, in combination with other medications
- Headaches, in combination with other medications

## Generic & Brand Names

### *Generic*

- Amobarbital
- Aprobarbital
- Butabarbital
- Butalbital
- Mephobarbital
- Metharbital
- Pentobarbital
- Phenobarbital
- Secobarbital
- Secobarbital and Amobarbital
- Talbutal

### *Brand*

- Alurate
- Amaphen

- Amytal
- Ancalixir
- Anolor-300
- Anoquan
- Arcet
- Axotal
- Azma Aid
- Bancap
- Barbita
- Bronkolixir
- Bronkotabs
- Bucet
- Busodium
- Butace
- Butalan
- Butalgen
- Butisol
- Cafergot PB
- Dolmar
- Endolor
- Esgic
- Esgic-Plus4
- Ezol
- Femcet
- Fiorgen PF
- Fioricet
- Fiorinal
- Fiormor
- Fortabs
- G-1
- Gemonil
- Isobutal
- Isocet
- Isolin
- Isollyl Improved
- Isopap

- Laniroif
- Lanorinal
- Luminal
- Marnal
- Mebaral
- Medigesic
- Mudrane GG
- Nembutal
- Nova-Rectal
- Novopentobarb
- Novosecobarb
- Pacaps
- Phrenilin
- Phrenilin Forte
- Primatene "P" Formula
- Repan
- Sarisol No. 2
- Seconal
- Sedapap
- Solfoton
- Tecnal
- Tencet
- Theodrine
- Theodrine Pediatric
- Theofed
- Triad
- Triaprin
- Tuinal
- Two-Dyne
- Vibutal

## Street Names

- Barbs
- Pheenies
- Red Birds
- Reds
- Tooies
- Yellow Jackets
- Yellows

## Signs & Symptoms

### Intoxication

- Slurred speech
- Disorientation
- Drunken behavior without odor of alcohol

### Overdose

- Weak tachycardia
- Shallow respiration
- Clammy skin
- Dilated pupils
- Coma

### Withdrawal

- Anxiety
- Insomnia
- Tremors
- Delirium
- Seizures
- Coma

## Psychotropic & Other Medication Reactions

### Anticonvulsants

- Seizure pattern changes

### Antihistamines *Guide 205*

- Dangerous sedation

### Beta-Blockers *Guide 211*

- Dangerous sedation

### Clozapine *Guide 220*

- Toxic to CNS

## Assessment

- Assess scene safety
  *Guide 402*
- Use PPE *Guide 002*
- Approach patient *Guide 003*
- Primary and secondary
  medical survey *Guide 403*
- Medications
- Brief mental status exam
  *Guide 404*

- Lethality assessment
  *Guide 407*
- Emotional first aid
  *Guide 004*

## Reporting

- Patient description
- Chief complaint
- Medical findings
- Mental status
- Lethality

## (GUIDE 305) BENZODIAZEPINES

### Description

- Tranquilizer
- Anticonvulsant
- Generic available
- Addictive

### Medical Uses *Guide 210*

- Anxiety Disorder
  *Guide 106*
- Dissociative Identity
  Disorder *Guide 114*
- Obsessive Compulsive
  Disorder *Guide 122*
- Panic Disorder *Guide 124*
- Personality Disorders
  *Guide 127*
- Phobias *Guide 129*
- Post-Traumatic Stress
  Disorder *Guide 130*
- Separation Anxiety
  Disorder *Guide 132*
- Alcohol withdrawal
  *Guide 302*
- Muscle spasms

- Seizure disorders
- Short-term insomnia

### Generic & Brand Names

*Generic*

- Alprazolam
- Bromazepam
- Chlordiazepoxide
- Clonazepam
- Clorazepate
- Diazepam
- Estrazolam
- Flurazepam
- Halazepam
- Ketazolam
- Lorazepam
- Midazolam
- Nitrazepam
- Oxazepam
- Prazepam
- Quazepam
- Temazepam

3

## Brand

- Alprazolam Intensol
- Apo-Alpraz
- Apo-Chlordiazepoxide
- Apo-Clorazepate
- Apo-Diazepam
- Apo-Flurazepam
- Apo-Lorazepam
- Apo-Oxazepam
- Ativan
- Centrax
- Clindex
- Clinoxide
- Dalmane
- Diastat
- Diazemuls
- Diazepam Intensol
- Doral
- Klonopin
- Lectopam
- Librax
- Libritabs
- Librium
- Lidoxide
- Limbitrol
- Limbitrol DS
- Lipoxide
- Loftran
- Lorazepam Intensol
- Medilium
- Meval
- Mogadon
- Novo-Alprazol
- Novoclopate
- Novodipam
- Novoflupam
- Novolorazem
- Novopoxide
- Novoxapam
- Nu-Alpraz
- Nu-Loraz
- Paxipam
- PMS Diazepam
- ProSom
- Restoril
- Rivotril
- Serax
- Solium
- Somnol
- T-Quil
- Tranxene
- Traxene-SD
- Traxene T-tab
- Valium
- Valrelease
- Vivol
- Xanax
- Zapex
- Zebrax
- Zetran

## Street Names

- Candy
- Tranks
- V
- Vitamin V
- Xany Bars

## Signs & Symptoms

### Intoxication

- Bradycardia
- Hypotension
- Nystagmus
- Slurred speech
- Incoordination
- Unsteady gait

- Difficulty focusing attention
- Memory impairment
- Impaired judgment

*Overdose*

- Bradycardia
- Hypotension
- Decreased respirations
- Nausea and/or vomiting
- Stupor
- Coma

*Withdrawal*

- Tachycardia
- Hypertension
- Increased respirations
- Hand tremor
- Insomnia
- Anxiety *Guide 106*
- Psychomotor agitation
- Transient visual, tactile, or auditory hallucinations
- Seizures

## Psychotropic & Other Medication Reactions

*Anticonvulsants*

- Change in seizure pattern

*Antidepressants — Tricyclic*
*Guide 203*

- Increased sedation

*Antihistamines Guide 205*

- Increased sedative effect of both drugs

*CNS Depressants*

- Increased sedative effect

*MAO Inhibitors Guide 231*

- Deep sedation
- Rage
- Seizures

## Other Interactions

*Alcohol Guide 302*

- Heavy sedation

*Marijuana Guide 318*

- Heavy sedation

## Assessment

- Assess scene safety *Guide 402*
- Use PPE *Guide 002*
- Approach patient *Guide 003*
- Primary and secondary medical survey *Guide 403*
- Medications
- Brief mental status exam *Guide 404*
- Brief psychosocial history *Guide 405*
- Emotional first aid *Guide 004*

## Reporting

- Patient description
- Chief complaint
- Medical findings
- Medications and compliance
- Known diagnoses
- Mental status
- Lethality
- Psychosocial history

### Description

- Sedative, hypnotic
- Generic available
- Highly addictive

### Medical Uses *Guide 217*

- Insomnia

### Generic & Brand Names

*Generic*

- Chloral Hydrate

*Brand*

- Aquachloral
- Notec
- Novochlorhydrate

### Street Names

- Coral
- Corals
- Christmas
- Christmas Rolls
- Mickey Finn
- Knock-Out Drops

### Signs & Symptoms

*Intoxication*

- Bradycardia
- Hypotension
- Nystagmus
- Slurred speech
- Incoordination
- Unsteady gait
- Difficulty focusing attention
- Memory impairment
- Impaired judgment

*Overdose*

- Bradycardia
- Hypotension
- Decreased respirations
- Nausea or vomiting
- Stupor
- Coma

*Withdrawal*

- Tachycardia
- Hypertension
- Increased respirations
- Hand tremors
- Insomnia
- Anxiety *Guide 106*
- Psychomotor agitation
- Transient visual, tactile, or auditory hallucinations
- Seizures

### Psychotropic & Other Medication Reactions

*Anticoagulants*

- Possible hemorrhaging

*Antidepressants — Tricyclic*
*Guide 203*

- Increased sedation

*Antihistamines Guide 205*

- Increased sedation

*Clozapine Guide 220*

- Toxic effect on CNS

*Guanfacine Guide 225*

- Increased sedation

3

*MAO Inhibitors* Guide 231

- Increased sedation

*Molindone* Guide 237

- Increased sedation

*Phenothiazines* Guide 245

- Increased sedation

*Selective Serotonin Reuptake Inhibitors (SSRIs)* Guide 249

- Increased sedation

## Other Interactions

*Alcohol* Guide 302

- Increased sedation

*Marijuana* Guide 318

- Severely impaired mental and physical functioning

## Assessment

- Assess scene safety Guide 402
- Use PPE Guide 002
- Approach patient Guide 003
- Primary and secondary medical survey Guide 403
- Medications
- Brief mental status exam Guide 404
- Emotional first aid Guide 004

## Reporting

- Patient description
- Chief complaint
- Medical findings
- Mental status
- Lethality

---

## GUIDE 307  COCAINE

### Description

- Naturally occurring substance produced by the coca plant
- Product may be consumed in a variety of refined forms
- Cocaine hydrochloride powder is typically "snorted" or injected
- Cocaine alkaloid (crack) is typically smoked
- Highly addictive

### Duration of Effect

- 5-30 minutes
- May be extended with repeated use

### Medical Uses

- Facial surgery
- Nasal surgery
- Oral surgery

## Street Names

- Blow
- Bump
- C
- Candy
- Charlie
- Coke
- Crack
- Flake
- Rock
- Snow
- Toot

## Signs & Symptoms

### Intoxication

- Tachycardia
- Hypertension
- Hyperthermia
- Pupil dilation
- Excessive perspiration
- Violent or erratic behavior
- Nausea or vomiting
- Psychomotor agitation
- Confusion
- Paranoia *Guide 125*

### Overdose

- Tachycardia
- Hypertension
- Hyperthermia
- Pupil dilation
- Excessive perspiration
- Seizure
- Coma
- Respiratory arrest
- Agitated delirium
- Stroke
- Heart attack

### Withdrawal

- Fatigue
- Vivid unpleasant dreams
- Insomnia or hypersomnia
- Increased appetite
- Agitation

## Medications Used in Treatment

*Antidepressants — Tricyclic Guide 203*

- Antidepressant
- Generic available
- Nonaddictive

## Psychotropic & Other Medication Reactions

*Amphetamines Guide 202*

- Dangerous stimulation of the nervous system

*Antidepressants — Tricyclic Guide 203*

- Increased chance of irregular heartbeat

*Antivirals — Influenza Guide 206*

- Dangerous overstimulation

*Beta-Blockers Guide 211*

- Cardiac arrhythmias
- Decreased effect of medication

*Carbidopa & Levodopa (Sinemet) Guide 216*

- Can increase cardiac dysrhythmia

**Clozapine (Clozaril)**
*Guide 220*

- Possible cardiac arrhythmias

**Ergoloid Mesylates** *Guide 223*

- Overstimulation

**Ergotamine, Belladonna, & Phenobarbital** *Guide 224*

- Excessive tachycardia

**Levodopa** *Guide 228*

- Risk of cardiac arrhythmias

**Lithium** *Guide 229*

- Possible psychosis

**Loxapine (Loxitane)**
*Guide 230*

- Can increase toxicity of both drugs

**MAO Inhibitors** *Guide 231*

- Potentially fatal excessive stimulation

**Maprotiline (Ludiomil)**
*Guide 232*

- Excessive intoxication

**Methylphenidate** *Guide 234*

- High risk of cardiac arrhythmias
- Hypertension

**Pergolide (Permax)** *Guide 244*

- Increased chance of adverse reactions

**Selegiline** *Guide 248*

- Hypertension
- Tachycardia

**Tolcapone (Tasmar)**
*Guide 252*

- Possible hallucinations

## Other Interactions

**Narcotic Drugs** *Guide 322*

- Increased toxic effect of cocaine

## Assessment

- Assess scene safety *Guide 402*
- Use PPE *Guide 002*
- Approach patient *Guide 003*
- Primary and secondary medical survey *Guide 403*
- Medications
- Brief mental status exam *Guide 404*
- Lethality assessment *Guide 407*
- Brief psychosocial history *Guide 405*
- Emotional first aid *Guide 004*

## Reporting

- Patient description
- Chief complaint
- Medical findings
- Mental status
- Lethality

## Description

- Narcotic Analgesic
- Generic available
- Highly addictive

## Medical Uses

- Cough suppressant
- Diarrhea treatment
- Pain relief

## Generic & Brand Names

### Generic

- Codeine
- Codeine and Terpin Hydrate

### Brand

- Actagen-C Cough
- Actifed with Codeine Cough
- Allerfrin with Codeine
- Ambay Cough
- Ambenyl Cough
- Ambophen Expectorant
- Aprodrine with Codeine
- Bayhistine DH
- Bayhistine Expectorant
- Baytussin AC
- Baytussin Expectorant
- Benylin with Codeine
- Bromanyl
- Brontex
- Calcidrine
- Calmylin with Codeine
- Cheracol
- CoActifed
- CoActifed Expectorant

- Codehist DH
- Codeine Sulfate
- Codimal PH
- Colrex Compound
- Coricidin with Codeine
- Cotridin
- Cotridin Expectorant
- C-Tussin Expectorant
- Decohistine DH
- Deproist Expectorant with Codeine
- Dihistine DH
- Dihistine Expectorant
- Expectorant with Codeine
- Glydeine Cough
- Guiatuss A.C.
- Guiatussin DAC
- Guiatussin with Codeine Liquid
- Histafed
- Isoclor Expectorant
- Mallergan-VC with Codeine
- Midahist DH
- Mytussin AC
- Mytussin DAC
- Nortussin with Codeine
- Novagest Expectorant with Codeine
- Novahistex C
- Novahistine DH Expectorant
- Novahistine DH Liquid
- Novahistine Expectorant
- Nucochem
- Nucochem Expectorant
- Nucochem Pediatric Expectorant

3

- Nucofed
- Nucofed Expectorant
- Nucofed Pediatric Expectorant
- Omni-Tuss
- Paveral
- Pediacof Cough
- Pediatuss Cough
- Penazine VC with Cough
- Phenameth VC with Codeine
- Phenergran VC with Codeine
- Phenergran with Codeine
- Phenhist DH with Codeine
- Phenhist Expectorant
- Pherazine VC with Codeine
- Pherazine with Codeine
- Promehist with Codeine
- Prometh VC with Codeine
- Prunicodeine
- Robafen AC Cough
- Robafen DAC
- Robitussin A-C
- Robitussin-DAC
- Rolatuss Expectorant
- Ryna-C Liquid
- Ryna-CX Liquid
- Soma Compound
- Statuss Expectorant
- Terpin Hydrate and Codeine Syrup
- Tolu-Sed Cough
- Triacin-C Cough
- Triafed with Codeine
- Tricodene #1
- Trifed-C Cough
- Tussar SF
- Tussar-2

- Tussirex with Codeine Liquid

## Street Names

- Captain Cody
- Cody
- Doors and Fours
- Loads
- Pancakes and Syrup
- Schoolboy

## Signs & Symptoms

### Intoxication

- Slow respiration
- Constricted pupils
- Euphoria
- Drowsiness
- Slurred speech
- Difficulty focusing attention
- Perceptual disturbances
- Impaired memory

### Overdose

- Pupil constriction
- Bradycardia
- Hypotension
- Decreased respirations
- Seizures
- Coma

### Withdrawal

- Watery eyes
- Runny nose
- Fatigue
- Irritability
- Loss of appetite
- Cold sweats
- Nausea and vomiting

- Severe cramps
- Tremors
- Panic *Guide 124*

## Psychotropic & Other Medication Reactions

*Analgesics*
- Increased analgesic effect

*Anticoagulants*
- Increased anticoagulant effect

*Antidepressants — Tricyclic Guide 203*
- Increased scdative effect

*Antihistamines Guide 205*
- Increased sedative effect

*Butorphanol*
- Possibly precipitates withdrawal with chronic narcotic use

*Carteolol*
- Dangerous sedation

*Cimetidine*
- Toxicity and possible increased narcotic effect

*Clozapine (Clozaril) Guide 220*
- Toxic effect on CNS

*Ethinamate*
- Dangerous increased effects of Ethinamate

*MAO Inhibitors Guide 231*
- Serious toxicity, potentially fatal

*Methyprylon*
- Increased sedative effect, possibly to dangerous level

*Nabilone*
- Greater depression of CNS

*Nalbuphine*
- Possibly precipitates withdrawal with chronic narcotic use

*Naltrexone Guide 239*
- Precipitates withdrawal symptoms
- Coma
- Respiratory arrest
- Death

*Nitrates*
- Excessive hypertension

*Pentazocine*
- Possibly precipitates withdrawal with chronic narcotic use

*Sedatives*
- Increased sedative effect

*Selegiline Guide 248*
- Severe toxicity
- Respiratory difficulty
- Seizures
- Coma

### Sleep Inducers
- Increased sedative effect

### Sotalol
- Dangerous sedation

### Selective Serotonin Reuptake Inhibitors (SSRIs) *Guide 249*
- Increased sedative effect

### Tramadol
- Increased sedation

### Tranquilizers
- Increased sedation

## Other Interactions

### Alcohol *Guide 302*
- Increased intoxicating effect of alcohol

### Cocaine *Guide 307*
- Increased toxic effect of cocaine

### Marijuana *Guide 318*
- Impaired physical and mental performance

## Assessment
- Assess scene safety *Guide 402*
- Use PPE *Guide 002*
- Approach patient *Guide 003*
- Primary and secondary medical survey *Guide 403*
- Medications
- Brief mental status exam *Guide 404*
- Lethality assessment *Guide 407*

## Reporting
- Patient description
- Chief complaint
- Medical findings
- Mental status
- Lethality

## GUIDE 309 — COUGH MEDICINE OTC (OVER THE COUNTER)

### Description
- Dextromethorphan
- Cough suppressant, antitussive
- Generic available
- Nonaddictive

### Medical Uses
- Cough suppressant

### Brand Names
- Coricidin HBP
- Delsym

- Drixoral
- Pertussin
- Robitussin
- Vicks Formula 44

## Street Names

- Dex
- DX
- Red Devils
- Robo
- Robo Fry
- Rojo
- Skittles
- Triple C's
- Tussin
- Vitamin D

## Signs & Symptoms

### *Intoxication*

- Hypertension
- Hyperthermia
- Flushing
- Excessive perspiration
- Itchy skin
- Dry mouth
- Hyperactivity

### *Overdose*

- Irregular heartbeat
- Shallow respirations
- Nausea and vomiting
- Abdominal pain
- Hallucinations
- Delusions
- Numbness of fingers and toes
- Stupor
- Seizures
- Coma

## Psychotropic & Other Medication Reactions

### *Doxepin* Guide 203

- Increased risk of toxicity for both drugs

### *MAO Inhibitors* Guide 231

- Hypotension
- Hyperthermia
- Disorientation
- Coma

### *Sedatives & Other CNS Depressants*

- Increased sedation

## Assessment

- Assess scene safety Guide 402
- Use PPE Guide 002
- Approach patient Guide 003
- Primary and secondary medical survey Guide 403
- Medications
- Brief mental status exam Guide 404
- Lethality assessment Guide 407
- Brief psychosocial history Guide 405

## Reporting

- Patient description
- Chief complaint
- Medical findings
- Mental status
- Lethality assessment
- Psychosocial history

## Description

- 3-4 Methylenedioxymeth-amphetamine
- Chemically similar to amphetamine and mescaline
- Stimulant, hallucinogen
- Taken orally

### Duration of Effect

- 4-6 hours per dose
- Multiple doses last 12 to 24 hours

## Street Names

- Adam
- Clarity
- Ecstasy
- Love pills
- Pills
- Roll or Rolling
- X
- XTC

## Signs & Symptoms

### Intoxication

- Increased heart rate
- Increased blood pressure
- Hyperthermia
- Hyperactivity
- Dehydration
- Euphoria
- Increased libido
- Mild hallucinogenic effects
- Dehydration

### Overdose

- Confusion
- Dangerous hyperthermia
- Heart attack
- Stroke
- Coma

## Psychotropic & Other Medication Reactions

### Antidepressants—Tricyclic Guide 203

- Decreased amphetamine effect

### Antihypertensives

- Decreased antihypertensive effect

### Beta-Blockers Guide 211

- Hypertension, bradycardia

### Carbonic Anhydrase Inhibitors

- Increased amphetamine effect

### CNS Stimulants

- Excessive CNS stimulation

### Furazolidone

- Sudden and severe hypertension

### Sympathomimetics

- Seizures

### Thyroid Hormones

- Cardiac arrhythmias

### Assessment

- Assess scene safety
  *Guide 402*
- Use PPE *Guide 002*
- Approach patient *Guide 003*
- Primary and secondary
  medical survey *Guide 403*
- Medications

- Brief mental status exam
  *Guide 404*
- Lethality assessment
  *Guide 407*

### Reporting

- Patient description
- Chief complaint
- Medical findings
- Mental status
- Lethality

---

## (GUIDE 311) FENTANYL

### Description

- Narcotic analgesic
- Generic available
- Highly addictive

### Medical Uses

- Pain relief

### Generic & Brand Names

*Generic*

- Fentanyl

*Brand*

- Actiq
- Duragesic

### Street Names

- Apache
- China Girl
- China White
- Dance Fever
- Friend
- Goodfella

- Jackpot
- Murder 8
- Tango and Cash
- TNT

### Signs & Symptoms

*Intoxication*

- Decreased respirations
- Constricted pupils
- Euphoria
- Drowsiness
- Slurred speech
- Difficulty focusing
  attention
- Perceptual disturbances
- Impaired memory

*Overdose*

- Pupil constriction
- Bradycardia
- Hypotension
- Decreased respirations
- Seizures
- Coma

## Withdrawal

- Watery eyes
- Runny nose
- Fatigue
- Irritability
- Loss of appetite
- Cold sweats
- Nausea and vomiting
- Severe cramps
- Tremors
- Panic *Guide 124*

## Psychotropic & Other Medication Reactions

### Analgesics

- Increased analgesic effect

### Anticoagulants

- Increased anticoagulant effect

### Antidepressants — Tricyclic
*Guide 203*

- Increased sedative effect

### Antihistamines *Guide 205*

- Increased sedative effect

### Butorphanol

- Possibly precipitates withdrawal with chronic narcotic use

### Carteolol

- Dangerous sedation

### Cimetidine

- Toxicity and possibly increased narcotic effect

### Clozapine *Guide 220*

- Toxic effect on CNS

### Ethinamate

- Dangerously increased effects of ethinamate

### MAO Inhibitors *Guide 231*

- Serious toxicity
- Potentially fatal

### Methyprylon

- Increased sedative effect, possibly to dangerous level

### Nabilone

- Greater depression of CNS

### Nalbuphine

- Possibly precipitates withdrawal with chronic narcotic use

### Naltrexone *Guide 239*

- Precipitates withdrawal symptoms
- Coma
- Respiratory arrest
- Death

### Nitrates

- Excessive hypertension

### Pentazocine

- Possibly precipitates withdrawal with chronic narcotic use

### Sedatives

- Increased sedative effect

### Selegiline *Guide 248*

- Severe toxicity, respiratory difficulty, seizures, coma

### Sleep Inducers

- Increased sedative effect

### Sotalol

- Dangerous sedation

### SSRIs *Guide 249*

- Increased sedative effect

### Tramadol

- Increased sedation

### Tranquilizers

- Increased sedation

## Other Interactions

### Alcohol *Guide 302*

- Increased intoxicating effect of alcohol

### Cocaine *Guide 307*

- Increased toxic effect of cocaine

### Marijuana *Guide 318*

- Impaired physical and mental performance

## Assessment

- Assess scene safety *Guide 402*
- Use PPE *Guide 002*
- Approach patient *Guide 003*
- Primary and secondary medical survey *Guide 403*
- Medications
- Brief mental status exam *Guide 404*
- Lethality assessment *Guide 407*
- Emotional first aid *Guide 004*

## Reporting

- Patient description
- Chief complaint
- Medical findings
- Mental status
- Lethality

## GUIDE 312  GHB

### Description

- Gamma-hydroxybutyrate
- CNS depressant
- Available as clear liquid, white powder, tablet, or capsule
- Effects begin in 10-20 minutes and typically last up to 4 hours
- Generally abused for its intoxicating, sedative, and euphoric properties

- Sometimes used by body-builders for its growth-hormone-releasing effects
- Sometimes used as a date rape drug

## Street Names

- G
- Georgia Home Boy
- Grievous Bodily Harm
- Liquid Ecstasy

## Signs & Symptoms

*Intoxication*

- Relaxation
- Sedation—drowsiness
- Bradycardia
- Hypotension
- Headache
- Euphoria
- Slowed respirations
- Drowsiness
- Enhanced sexual performance

*Overdose*

- Nausea and/or vomiting
- Headache
- Loss of reflexes
- Bradycardia

- Slow, shallow respirations
- Coma

*Note: GHB is cleared from the body relatively quickly, so it is sometimes difficult to detect in emergency departments.*

## Psychotropic & Other Medication Reactions

- Unknown

## Assessment

- Assess scene safety *Guide 402*
- Use PPE *Guide 002*
- Approach patient *Guide 003*
- Primary and secondary medical survey *Guide 403*
- Medications
- Brief mental status exam *Guide 404*
- Emotional first aid *Guide 004*

## Reporting

- Patient description
- Chief complaint
- Medical findings
- Mental status

## (GUIDE 313) HASHISH

## Description

- Delta-9-tetrahydrocannabi-nol (THC)-rich, resinous material from cannabis plants

- Variety of forms: balls, cakes, or cookie-like sheets
- THC can be extracted as a viscous amber oil
- Usually smoked; sometimes ingested

## Street Names

- Boom
- Hash
- Hash Oil
- Hemp

## Signs & Symptoms

### Intoxication

- Euphoria
- Impaired motor coordination
- Decreased social inhibition
- Increased appetite
- Short-term memory impairment
- Difficulty concentrating
- Altered sensory perception
- Impaired judgment

### Overdose

- Paranoia *Guide 125*
- Hallucinations
- Social withdrawal

## Psychotropic & Other Medication Reactions

*Amphetamines Guide 202*

- Frequent use severely impairs mental functioning

*Antidepressants — Tricyclic Guide 203*

- Excessive drowsiness
- Increased risk of side effects

*Antihistamines Guide 205*

- Increased sedation

*Barbiturates Guide 209*

- Excessive sedation

*Benzodiazepines Guide 210*

- Heavy sedation

*Beta-Blockers Guide 211*

- Possible hypertension

*Bromocriptine Guide 212*

- Increased fatigue
- Lethargy
- Fainting

*Carbamazepine (Tegretol) Guide 215*

- Increased possibility of adverse effects of this drug

*Carbidopa & Levodopa (Sinemet) Guide 216*

- Increased lethargy
- Fatigue
- Fainting

*Clozapine (Clozaril) Guide 220*

- Possible cardiac arrhythmias

*Ergotamine, Belladonna, & Phenobarbital Guide 224*

- Possible oversedation
- Drowsiness

3

*Haloperidol (Haldol)*
Guide 226
- Frequent use may result in toxic psychosis

*Lithium* Guide 229
- Possible psychosis
- Increased tremor activity

*Loxapine (Loxitane)*
Guide 230
- Can increase toxicity of both drugs

*MAO Inhibitors* Guide 231
- Overstimulation

*Maprotiline (Ludiomil)*
Guide 232
- Excessive drowsiness

*Meprobamate* Guide 233
- Increased sedative effects of meprobamate

*Molindone (Moban)*
Guide 237
- Increased drowsiness

*Orphenadrine* Guide 242
- Increased drowsiness
- Dry mouth
- Fainting
- Muscular weakness

*Phenothiazines* Guide 245
- Drowsiness
- Increased antinausea effect

*Selegiline* Guide 248
- Tachycardia

*SSRIs* Guide 249
- Excessive drowsiness
- Increased risk of side effects

*Thiothixene (Navane)*
Guide 251
- Possible fainting with frequent use
- Psychosis

*Tolcapone (Tasmar)*
Guide 252
- Possible hallucinations

*Trazodone* Guide 253
- May increase heartbeat irregularities

## Assessment

- Assess scene safety Guide 402
- Use PPE Guide 002
- Approach patient Guide 003
- Primary and secondary medical survey Guide 403
- Medications
- Brief mental status exam Guide 404
- Lethality assessment Guide 407
- Emotional first aid Guide 004

## Reporting

- Patient description
- Chief complaint
- Medical findings
- Mental status
- Lethality

## GUIDE 314 HEROIN

### Description

- Semisynthetic narcotic
- Injected, smoked, snorted
- Highly addictive

### Street Names

- Brown Sugar
- Dope
- H
- Horse
- Junk
- Skunk
- Smack
- Tits
- White Horse

### Signs & Symptoms

*Intoxication*

- Slowed respirations
- Constricted pupils
- Euphoria
- Drowsiness
- Slurred speech
- Difficulty focusing attention
- Perceptual disturbances
- Impaired memory

*Overdose*

- Bradycardia
- Hypotension
- Decreased respirations
- Pupil constriction
- Seizures
- Coma

*Withdrawal*

- Watery eyes
- Runny nose
- Fatigue
- Irritability
- Loss of appetite
- Cold sweats
- Nausea and vomiting
- Severe cramps
- Tremors
- Panic *Guide 124*

### Psychotropic & Other Medication Reactions

*Analgesics*

- Increased analgesic effect

*Anticoagulants*

- Increased anticoagulant effect

*Antidepressants — Tricyclic*
*Guide 203*

- Increased sedative effect

*Antihistamines Guide 205*

- Increased sedative effect

### Butorphanol
- Possibly precipitates withdrawal with chronic narcotic use

### Carteolol
- Dangerous sedation

### Cimetidine
- Toxicity
- Possibly increased narcotic effect

### Clozapine (Clozaril)
Guide 220
- Toxic effect on CNS

### Ethinamate
- Dangerous increased effects of ethinamate

### MAO Inhibitors Guide 231
- Serious toxicity, potentially fatal

### Methyprylon
- Increased sedative effect, possibly to dangerous level

### Nabilone
- Greater depression of CNS

### Nalbuphine
- Possibly precipitates withdrawal with chronic narcotic use

### Naltrexone Guide 239
- Precipitates withdrawal symptoms

### Coma
- Respiratory arrest
- Death

### Nitrates
- Excessive hypertension

### Pentazocine
- Possibly precipitates withdrawal with chronic narcotic use

### Sedatives
- Increased sedative effect

### Selegiline Guide 248
- Severe toxicity
- Respiratory difficulty
- Seizures
- Coma

### Sleep Inducers
- Increased sedative effect

### Sotalol
- Dangerous sedation

### SSRIs Guide 249
- Increased sedative effect

### Tramadol
- Increased sedation

### Tranquilizers
- Increased sedation

## Other Interactions

*Alcohol Guide 302*

- Increased intoxicating effect of alcohol

*Cocaine Guide 307*

- Increased toxic effect of cocaine

*Marijuana Guide 318*

- Impaired physical and mental performance

## Assessment

- Assess scene safety *Guide 402*
- Use PPE *Guide 002*
- Approach patient *Guide 003*

- Primary and secondary medical survey *Guide 403*
- Medications
- Brief mental status exam *Guide 404*
- Lethality assessment *Guide 407*
- Emotional first aid *Guide 004*

## Reporting

- Patient description
- Chief complaint
- Medical findings
- Mental status
- Lethality

3

---

## (GUIDE 315) INHALANTS

### Description

Chemically diverse group of psychoactive substances commonly found in:

- Adhesives and glues
- Aerosol propellant
- Cleaning fluids
- Lighter fluid: butane, propane
- Nitrites
- Nitrous Oxide
- Paint products
- Solvents: paint thinners, gasoline

### *Duration of Effect*

Typically inhaled through nose and/or mouth
- 15-45 minutes for solvents and paints
- 30 seconds to 30 minutes for Nitrites
- 1-2 minutes for Nitrous Oxide

### Medical Uses

- Amyl Nitrate used for angina pectoris
- Nitrous Oxide used as a dental anesthetic

## Street Names

- Air Blast
- Bagging
- Discorama
- Hippie Crack
- Laughing Gas
- Locker Room
- Moon Gas
- Nitrous
- Oz
- Rush
- Satan's Secret
- Texas Shoe Shine
- Whippets

## Signs & Symptoms

*Intoxication*

- Dizziness
- Nystagmus
- Incoordination
- Slurred speech
- Unsteady gait
- Lethargy
- Depressed reflexes
- Psychomotor retardation
- Perceptual disturbances

*Overdose*

- Nausea and vomiting

- Severe cramps
- Decreased respiration, wheezing
- Cardiac arrhythmias
- Tremor
- Stupor
- Coma
- Sudden death

## Assessment

- Assess scene safety *Guide 402*
- Use PPE *Guide 002*
- Approach patient *Guide 003*
- Primary and secondary medical survey *Guide 403*
- Medications
- Brief mental status exam *Guide 404*
- Lethality assessment *Guide 407*
- Emotional first aid *Guide 004*

## Reporting

- Patient description
- Chief complaint
- Medical findings
- Mental status
- Lethality

## GUIDE 316 KETAMINE

### Description

- Dissociative anesthetic
- Approved for human use in medical settings
- Used widely in veterinary medicine

- Available as a liquid or white powder
- Often ingested or smoked with marijuana or tobacco; can be injected

## Medical Use

- Anesthetic

## Street Names

- Cat Valiums
- K
- Special K
- Vitamin K

## Signs & Symptoms

*Intoxication*

- Hypertension
- Tachycardia
- Slowed respiration
- Dream-like state
- Loss of coordination
- Difficulty focusing attention
- Memory impairments

*Overdose*

- Hypertension
- Tachycardia
- Hallucinations
- Amnesia *Guide 105*

- Delirium *Guide 111*
- Coma
- Respiratory arrest

## Assessment

- Assess scene safety *Guide 402*
- Use PPE *Guide 002*
- Approach patient *Guide 003*
- Primary and secondary medical survey *Guide 403*
- Medications
- Brief mental status exam *Guide 404*
- Lethality assessment *Guide 407*
- Emotional first aid *Guide 004*

## Reporting

- Patient description
- Chief complaint
- Medical findings
- Mental status
- Lethality

3

## ( GUIDE 317 ) LSD

## Description

- Lysergic acid diethylamide
- Synthetic
- Hallucinogen
- Most commonly available on blotter paper; also sold in tablet, capsule, and liquid forms
- Usually ingested; liquid sometimes dropped in eyes or absorbed sublingually

## Street Names

- Acid
- Cubes
- Fry
- Micro
- Microdot
- Sid
- Sunshine

## Signs & Symptoms

*Intoxication*

- Tachycardia
- Hypertension
- Hyperthermia
- Dilated pupils
- Increased blood sugar
- Perceptual distortions

*Overdose*

- Tachycardia
- Hypertension
- Hyperthermia
- Dilated pupils
- Increased blood sugar
- Perceptual distortions
- Intense hallucinations
- Paranoia *Guide 125*
- Psychosis

*Withdrawal*

- Flashbacks

## Assessment

- Assess scene safety *Guide 402*
- Use PPE *Guide 002*
- Approach patient *Guide 003*
- Primary and secondary medical survey *Guide 403*
- Medications
- Brief mental status exam *Guide 404*
- Lethality assessment *Guide 407*
- Emotional first aid *Guide 004*

## Reporting

- Patient description
- Chief complaint
- Medical findings
- Medications and compliance
- Known diagnoses
- Mental status
- Lethality

---

## (GUIDE 318) MARIJUANA

### Description

- Psychoactive substance derived from the cannabis plant
- Usually smoked
- May also be ingested

### Duration of Effect

- 1-4 hours

### Medical Uses (Not Approved Universally)

- HIV/AIDS
- Cancer
- Glaucoma
- Pain

### Street Names

- Blunt
- Chronic

- Dank
- Dope
- Ganja
- Green
- Herb
- Kind
- Pot
- Redge
- Weed

## Signs & Symptoms

### Intoxication

- Tachycardia
- Conjunctival injection (bloodshot eyes)
- Dry mouth
- Drowsiness
- Euphoria
- Slowed sensation of time
- Impaired motor coordination
- Decreased social inhibition
- Increased appetite
- Short-term memory impairment
- Difficulty concentrating
- Altered sensory perception
- Impaired judgment

### Overdose

- Paranoia *Guide 125*
- Hallucinations
- Social withdrawal

## Psychotropic & Other Medication Reactions

### Amphetamines *Guide 202*

- Frequent use severely impairs mental function

### Antidepressants—Tricyclic *Guide 203*

- Excessive drowsiness
- Increased risk of side effects

### Antihistamines *Guide 205*

- Increased sedation

### Barbiturates *Guide 209*

- Excessive sedation

### Benzodiazepines *Guide 210*

- Heavy sedation

### Beta-Blockers *Guide 211*

- Possible hypertension

### Bromocriptine *Guide 212*

- Increased fatigue
- Lethargy
- Fainting

### Carbamazepine (Tegretol) *Guide 215*

- Increased possibility of adverse effects of this drug

### Carbidopa & Levodopa (Sinemet) *Guide 216*

- Increased lethargy
- Fatigue
- Fainting

3

### Clozapine (Clozaril)
Guide 220
- Possible cardiac arrhythmias

### Ergotamine, Belladonna, & Phenobarbital Guide 224
- Possible oversedation, drowsiness

### Haloperidol (Haldol)
Guide 226
- Frequent use may result in toxic psychosis

### Lithium Guide 229
- Possible psychosis
- Increased tremor activity

### Loxapine (Loxitane)
Guide 230
- Can increase toxicity of both drugs

### MAO Inhibitors Guide 231
- Overstimulation

### Maprotiline (Ludiomil)
Guide 232
- Excessive drowsiness

### Meprobamate Guide 233
- Increased sedative effects of Meprobamate

### Molindone (Moban)
Guide 237
- Increased drowsiness

### Orphenadrine Guide 242
- Increased drowsiness
- Dry mouth
- Fainting
- Muscular weakness

### Phenothiazines Guide 245
- Drowsiness
- Increased antinausea effect

### Selegiline Guide 248
- Tachycardia

### SSRIs Guide 249
- Excessive drowsiness
- Increased risk of side effects

### Thiothixene (Navane)
Guide 251
- With frequent use, possible fainting
- Psychosis

### Tolcapone (Tasmar)
Guide 252
- Possible hallucinations

### Trazodone Guide 253
- May increase cardiac arrhythmias

## Assessment
- Assess scene safety Guide 402
- Use PPE Guide 002
- Approach patient Guide 003
- Primary and secondary medical survey Guide 403
- Medications

- Brief mental status exam
  *Guide 404*
- Brief psychosocial history
  *Guide 405*
- Emotional first aid
  *Guide 004*

## Reporting

- Patient description
- Chief complaint
- Medical findings
- Mental status
- Lethality
- Psychosocial history

## GUIDE 319 — MESCALINE & PEYOTE

### Description

- Peyote is a small, spineless cactus that grows in the Southwestern United States and Northern Mexico
- Often used by Native Americans in the Southwestern United States in religious ceremonies
- Mescaline can be extracted from the peyote cactus or produced synthetically
- Hallucinogen
- Can be ingested or smoked

### Street Names

- Buttons
- Cactus
- Mesc
- Mescal
- Mescaline
- Peyote

### Signs & Symptoms

*Intoxication*

- Tachycardia
- Hypertension
- Hyperthermia
- Dilated pupils
- Increased blood sugar
- Perceptual distortions

*Overdose*

- Tachycardia
- Hypertension
- Hyperthermia
- Dilated pupils
- Increased blood sugar
- Perceptual distortions
- Intense hallucinations
- Paranoia *Guide 125*
- Psychosis

*Withdrawal*

- Flashbacks

### Assessment

- Assess scene safety
  *Guide 402*
- Use PPE *Guide 002*
- Approach patient *Guide 003*
- Primary and secondary medical survey *Guide 403*
- Medications
- Brief mental status exam
  *Guide 404*
- Lethality assessment
  *Guide 407*

3

- Emotional first aid
  *Guide 004*

## Reporting
- Patient description
- Chief complaint

- Medical findings
- Medications and compliance
- Known diagnoses
- Mental status
- Lethality

## ( GUIDE 320 ) MORPHINE

### Description
- Narcotic analgesic
- Generic available
- Highly addictive

### Medical Use
- Pain relief

### Generic & Brand Names

*Generic*
- Morphine

*Brand*
- Astramorph
- Astramorph PF
- Avinza
- Duramorph
- Epimorph
- Kadian
- Morphitec
- M.O.S.
- M.O.S.-S.R.
- MS Contin
- MSIR
- MST Continus
- Oramorph
- Oramorph-SR
- RMS Uniserts

- Roxanol
- Roxanol SR
- Statex

### Street Names
- M
- Miss Emma
- Monkey
- Morph
- White Stuff

### Signs & Symptoms

*Intoxication*
- Slow respirations
- Constricted pupils
- Euphoria
- Drowsiness
- Slurred speech
- Difficulty focusing attention
- Perceptual disturbances
- Impaired memory

*Overdose*
- Pupil constriction
- Bradycardia
- Hypotension
- Decreased respirations
- Seizures
- Coma

3

### Withdrawal

- Watery eyes
- Runny nose
- Fatigue
- Irritability
- Loss of appetite
- Cold sweats
- Nausea and vomiting
- Severe cramps
- Tremors
- Panic *Guide 124*

## Psychotropic & Other Medication Reactions

### Analgesics

- Increased analgesic effect

### Anticoagulants

- Increased anticoagulant effect

### Antidepressants — Tricyclic
*Guide 203*

- Increased sedative effect

### Antihistamines *Guide 205*

- Increased sedative effect

### Butorphanol

- Possibly precipitates withdrawal with chronic narcotic use

### Carteolol

- Dangerous sedation

### Cimetidine

- Toxicity and possibly increased narcotic effect

### Clozapine (Clozaril)
*Guide 220*

- Toxic effect on CNS

### Ethinamate

- Dangerously increased effects of Ethinamate

### MAO Inhibitors *Guide 231*

- Serious toxicity
- Potentially fatal

### Methyprylon

- Increased sedative effect, possibly to dangerous level

### Nabilone

- Greater depression of CNS

### Nalbuphine

- Possibly precipitates withdrawal with chronic narcotic use

### Naltrexone *Guide 239*

- Precipitates withdrawal symptoms
- Coma
- Respiratory arrest
- Death

### Nitrates

- Excessive hypertension

3

### Pentazocine

- Possibly precipitates withdrawal with chronic narcotic use

### Sedatives

- Increased sedative effect

### Selegiline *Guide 248*

- Severe toxicity
- Respiratory difficulty
- Seizures
- Coma

### Sleep Inducers

- Increased sedative effect

### Sotalol

- Dangerous sedation

### SSRIs *Guide 249*

- Increased sedative effect

### Tramadol

- Increased sedation

### Tranquilizers

- Increased sedation

## Other Interactions

### Alcohol *Guide 302*

- Increased intoxicating effect of alcohol

### Cocaine *Guide 307*

- Increased toxic effect of cocaine

### Marijuana *Guide 318*

- Impaired physical and mental performance

## Assessment

- Assess scene safety *Guide 402*
- Use PPE *Guide 002*
- Approach patient *Guide 003*
- Primary and secondary medical survey *Guide 403*
- Medications
- Brief mental status exam *Guide 404*
- Lethality assessment *Guide 407*
- Emotional first aid *Guide 004*

## Reporting

- Patient description
- Chief complaint
- Medical findings
- Mental status
- Lethality

## Description

- Psilocybin and psilocin are the intoxicating agents found in mushrooms
- Both chemicals are obtained from certain mushrooms that grow in Mexico and Central America
- Hallucinogen
- Ingested; sometimes smoked

## Street Names

- Boomers
- Magic Mushrooms
- Purple Passion
- Shrooms

## Signs & Symptoms

*Intoxication*

- Tachycardia
- Hypertension
- Hyperthermia
- Dilated pupils
- Increased blood sugar
- Perceptual distortions

*Overdose*

- Tachycardia
- Hypertension
- Hyperthermia
- Dilated pupils

- Increased blood sugar
- Perceptual distortions
- Intense hallucinations
- Paranoia *Guide 125*
- Psychosis
- Kidney failure

*Withdrawal*

- Flashbacks

## Assessment

- Assess scene safety *Guide 402*
- Use PPE *Guide 002*
- Approach patient *Guide 003*
- Primary and secondary medical survey *Guide 403*
- Medications
- Brief mental status exam *Guide 404*
- Lethality assessment *Guide 407*
- Emotional first aid *Guide 004*

## Reporting

- Patient description
- Chief complaint
- Medical findings
- Medications and compliance
- Known diagnoses
- Mental status
- Lethality

## Description

- Narcotic analgesics
- Generic available
- Addictive

## Medical Uses

- Pain relief

## Generic & Brand Names

*Generic*

- Hydrocodone
- Hydrocodone and Acetaminophen
- Meperidine and Acetaminophen
- Oxycodone
- Oxycodone and Acetaminophen
- Propoxyphene
- Propoxyphene and Acetaminophen

*Brand*

- Anamine HD
- Anaplex HD
- Chlorgest-HD
- Citra Forte
- Codiclear DH
- Codimal DH
- Co-Gesic
- Coristex-DH
- Coristine-DH
- Darvocet
- Darvocet-N 100
- Darvocet-N 50
- Darvon

- Darvon-N
- Demerol-APA
- Dolene AP-65
- Duocet
- Endocet
- Hycodan
- Lorcet
- Lortab
- Oxycocet
- Oxycontin SR
- Percocet
- Percocet-Demi
- Pro Pox with APAP
- Roxicet
- Roxicodone
- Roxilox
- Tylox
- Tyrodone
- Ugesic
- Ultragesic
- Vanacet
- Vapocet
- Vicodin
- Wygesic

## Street Names

- Blues
- Happy Pills
- Hillbilly Heroin
- Kickers
- Oxy
- Oxy-Cotton
- Pain Killers
- Perks
- Rocks
- Vikes

## Signs & Symptoms

### Intoxication

- Slow respirations
- Constricted pupils
- Euphoria
- Drowsiness
- Slurred speech
- Difficulty focusing attention
- Perceptual disturbances
- Impaired memory

### Overdose

- Pupil constriction
- Bradycardia
- Hypotension
- Decreased respirations
- Seizures
- Coma

### Withdrawal

- Watery eyes
- Runny nose
- Fatigue
- Irritability
- Loss of appetite
- Cold sweats
- Nausea and/or vomiting
- Severe cramps
- Tremors
- Panic *Guide 124*

## Psychotropic & Other Medication Reactions

### Analgesics

- Increased analgesic effect

### Anticoagulants

- Increased anticoagulant effect

### Antidepressants — Tricyclic
*Guide 203*

- Increased sedative effect

### Antihistamines *Guide 205*

- Increased sedative effect

### Butorphanol

- Possibly precipitates withdrawal with chronic narcotic use

### Carteolol

- Dangerous sedation

### Cimetidine

- Toxicity and possible increased narcotic effect

### Clozapine (Clozaril)
*Guide 220*

- Toxic effect on CNS

### Ethinamate

- Dangerous increased effects of ethinamate

### MAO Inhibitors *Guide 231*

- Serious toxicity
- Potentially fatal

### Methyprylon

- Increased sedative effect, possibly to dangerous level

## Nabilone

- Greater depression of CNS

## Nalbuphine

- Possibly precipitates withdrawal with chronic narcotic use

## Naltrexone *Guide 239*

- Precipitates withdrawal symptoms
- Coma
- Respiratory arrest
- Death

## Nitrates

- Excessive hypertension

## Pentazocine

- Possibly precipitates withdrawal with chronic narcotic use

## Sedatives

- Increased sedative effect

## Selegiline *Guide 248*

- Severe toxicity
- Respiratory difficulty
- Seizure
- Coma

## Sleep Inducers

- Increased sedative effect

## Sotalol

- Dangerous sedation

## SSRIs *Guide 249*

- Increased sedative effect

## Tramadol

- Increased sedation

## Tranquilizers

- Increased sedation

## Other Interactions

### Alcohol *Guide 302*

- Increased intoxicating effect of alcohol

### Cocaine *Guide 307*

- Increased toxic effect of cocaine

### Marijuana *Guide 318*

- Impaired physical and mental performance

## Assessment

- Assess scene safety *Guide 402*
- Use PPE *Guide 002*
- Approach patient *Guide 003*
- Primary and secondary medical survey *Guide 403*
- Medications
- Brief mental status exam *Guide 404*
- Lethality assessment *Guide 407*
- Emotional first aid *Guide 004*

## Reporting

- Patient description
- Chief complaint
- Medical findings
- Mental status
- Lethality

# (GUIDE 323) OPIUM

## Description

- Narcotic analgesic
- Comes from the poppy Papaver somniferum
- Highly addictive
- Smoked, swallowed, sometimes injected

## Medical Use

- Pain relief

## Generic & Brand Names

### Generic

- Opium

### Brand

- Laudanum
- Pantopon

## Street Names

- Big O
- Black Stuff
- Block
- Gum
- Hop

## Signs & Symptoms

### Intoxication

- Slow respiration
- Constricted pupils
- Euphoria
- Drowsiness
- Slurred speech
- Difficulty focusing attention
- Perceptual disturbances
- Impaired memory

### Overdose

- Pupil constriction
- Bradycardia
- Hypotension
- Decreased respirations
- Seizures
- Coma

### Withdrawal

- Watery eyes
- Runny nose
- Fatigue
- Irritability
- Loss of appetite
- Cold sweats
- Nausea and/or vomiting
- Severe cramps
- Tremors
- Panic *Guide 124*

## Psychotropic & Other Medication Reactions

### Analgesics

- Increased analgesic effect

### Anticoagulants

- Increased anticoagulant effect

### Antidepressants — Tricyclic
*Guide 203*

- Increased sedative effect

### Antihistamines *Guide 205*

- Increased sedative effect

3

### Butorphanol

- Possibly precipitates withdrawal with chronic narcotic use

### Carteolol

- Dangerous sedation

### Cimetidine

- Toxicity and possibly increased narcotic effect

### Clozapine (Clozaril)
Guide 220

- Toxic effect on CNS

### Ethinamate

- Dangerously increased effects of ethinamate

### MAO Inhibitors Guide 231

- Serious toxicity
- Potentially fatal

### Methyprylon

- Increased sedative effect, possibly to dangerous level

### Nabilone

- Greater depression of CNS

### Nalbuphine

- Possibly precipitates withdrawal with chronic narcotic use

### Naltrexone Guide 239

- Precipitates withdrawal symptoms
- Coma

### Respiratory arrest
- Death

### Nitrates

- Excessive hypertension

### Pentazocine

- Possibly precipitates withdrawal with chronic narcotic use

### Sedatives

- Increased sedative effect

### Selegiline Guide 248

- Severe toxicity
- Respiratory difficulty
- Seizures
- Coma

### Sleep Inducers

- Increased sedative effect

### Sotalol

- Dangerous sedation

### SSRIs Guide 249

- Increased sedative effect

### Tramadol

- Increased sedation

### Tranquilizers

- Increased sedation

## Other Interactions

### Alcohol Guide 302

- Increased intoxicating effect of alcohol

**Cocaine** *Guide 307*

- Increased toxic effect of cocaine

**Marijuana** *Guide 318*

- Impaired physical and mental performance

## Assessment

- Assess scene safety *Guide 402*
- Use PPE *Guide 002*
- Approach patient *Guide 003*
- Primary and secondary medical survey *Guide 403*

- Medications
- Brief mental status exam *Guide 404*
- Lethality assessment *Guide 407*
- Emotional first aid *Guide 004*

## Reporting

- Patient description
- Chief complaint
- Medical findings
- Mental status
- Lethality

3

## GUIDE 324 PHENCYCLIDINE (PCP)

## Description

- Dissociative anesthetic and hallucinogen
- Previously used in veterinary medicine
- Not approved for human or animal use
- Swallowed, smoked, or injected

## Street Names

- Angel Dust
- Boat
- Embalming Fluid
- Hog
- Love Boat
- Peace Pill
- Rocket Fuel

## Signs & Symptoms

*Intoxication*

- Bradycardia
- Hypotension
- Nystagmus
- Numbness or diminished response to pain
- Blank stare
- Slurred speech
- Loss of coordination

*Overdose*

- Bradycardia
- Hypotension
- Auditory hallucinations
- Paranoia *Guide 125*
- Violent hostility

- Hyperacusis—painful sensitivity to sounds
- Psychosis
- Decreased respirations
- Coma

## Assessment

- Assess scene safety *Guide 402*
- Use PPE *Guide 002*
- Approach patient *Guide 003*
- Primary and secondary medical survey *Guide 403*

- Medications
- Brief mental status exam *Guide 404*
- Lethality assessment *Guide 407*
- Emotional first aid *Guide 004*

## Reporting

- Patient description
- Chief complaint
- Medical findings
- Mental status

---

# (GUIDE 325) RITALIN

## Description

- CNS stimulant
- Generic available
- Addictive

## Medical Uses *Guide 234*

- Attention Deficit Disorder *Guide 103*
- Adult depression *Guide 113*
- Narcolepsy *Guide 121*

## Generic & Brand Names

### *Generic*

- Methylphenidate
- Dexmethylphenidate

### *Brand*

- Concerta
- Focalin
- Metadate CD
- Metadate ER

- Methylin ER
- Ritalin
- Ritalin LA
- Ritalin SR

## Street Names

- Kibbles and Bits
- R-Ball
- Round Ball
- Speed
- Vitamin R
- West Coast

## Signs & Symptoms

### *Intoxication*

- Tachycardia
- Dilated pupils
- Elevated blood pressure
- Psychomotor agitation
- Muscular tension
- Euphoria

### Overdose

- Tachycardia
- Lowered blood pressure
- Decreased respirations
- Chest pain
- Cardiac arrhythmias
- Dystonia and muscular weakness
- Confusion
- Dyskinesia (deficits in voluntary movement)
- Seizure
- Coma
- Excessive strength

### Withdrawal

- Dysphoric mood; depression *Guide 113*
- Fatigue
- Vivid, unpleasant dreams
- Insomnia or hypersomnia
- Increased appetite
- Headache

## Psychotropic & Other Medication Reactions

### Anticholinergics

- Increased anticholinergic effect

### Anticoagulants—Oral

- Increased anticoagulant effect

### Anticonvulsants

- Increased anticonvulsant effect
- Decreased stimulant effect

### Antidepressants—Tricyclic
*Guide 203*

- Increased antidepressant effect
- Decreased stimulant effect

### Antihypertensives

- Decreased antihypertensive effect

### CNS Stimulants

- Overstimulation

### Dextrothyroxine

- Increased stimulation

### MAO Inhibitors *Guide 231*

- Dangerous hypertension

## Other Interactions

### Caffeine

- Hypertension

### Cocaine *Guide 307*

- Cardiac arrhythmias
- Hypertension

## Assessment

- Assess scene safety *Guide 402*
- Use PPE *Guide 002*
- Approach patient *Guide 003*
- Primary and secondary medical survey *Guide 403*
- Medications
- Brief mental status exam *Guide 404*
- Lethality assessment *Guide 407*

## Reporting

- Patient description
- Chief complaint
- Medical findings
- Medications and compliance
- Known diagnoses
- Mental status
- Lethality

---

## (GUIDE 326) ROHYPNOL (FLUNITRAZEPAM)

### Description

- Benzodiazepine *Guide 210*
- Not approved for prescription use in the United States
- Tablet or white powder
- Swallowed; sometimes snorted
- Dissolves easily in carbonated beverages

### Street Names

- Forget-Me Pill
- Mexican Valium
- R2
- Roche
- Roofies
- Roofinol
- Rope

### Signs & Symptoms

*Intoxication*

- Bradycardia
- Hypotension
- Decreased respirations
- Excessive sedation
- Urinary retention
- Anterograde Amnesia: memory loss during drug's effect

*Overdose*

- Bradycardia
- Hypotension
- Decreased respirations
- Nausea and/or vomiting
- Stupor
- Coma
- Respiratory arrest

### Psychotropic & Other Medication Reactions

*Anticonvulsants*

- Change in seizure pattern

*Antidepressants — Tricyclic Guide 203*

- Increased sedation

*Antihistamines Guide 205*

- Increased sedative effect of both drugs

*CNS Depressants*

- Increased sedative effect

*MAO Inhibitors Guide 231*

- Seizures, deep sedation, rage

*SSRIs Guide 249*

- Increased sedation

## Other Interactions

**Alcohol** *Guide 302*

- Heavy sedation

**Marijuana** *Guide 318*

- Heavy sedation

## Assessment

- Assess scene safety
  *Guide 402*
- Use PPE *Guide 002*
- Approach patient *Guide 003*
- Primary and secondary
  medical survey *Guide 403*

- Medications
- Brief mental status exam
  *Guide 404*
- Lethality assessment
  *Guide 407*
- Emotional first aid
  *Guide 004*

## Reporting

- Patient description
- Chief complaint
- Medical findings
- Mental status
- Lethality

---

## (GUIDE 327) SOMA

**3**

## Description

- Muscle relaxant
- Generic available
- Possibly addictive
- Taken orally in pill or
  tablet form

## Medical Use

- Muscle spasms

## Generic & Brand Names

*Generic*

- Carisoprodol

*Brand*

- Rela
- Sodol
- Soma
- Soma Compound with
  Codeine

- Sopridol
- Soridol

## Street Names

- D's Dance
- Dan's
- DAN5513
- Dance
- Dannies
- Soma

## Signs & Symptoms

*Intoxication*

- Tachycardia
- Facial flushing
- Incoordination
- Dizziness
- Drowsiness

### Overdose

- Nausea and/or vomiting
- Headache
- Diarrhea
- Shaking and tremors
- Severe weakness
- Sensation of paralysis
- Difficulty breathing
- Coma

### Withdrawal

- Headache
- Insomnia
- Chills
- Nausea and vomiting
- Abdominal cramps

## Psychotropic & Other Medication Reactions

### Antidepressants — Tricyclic
*Guide 203*

- Increased sedation

### Antihistamines *Guide 205*

- Increased sedation

### Clozapine (Clozaril)
*Guide 220*

- Toxic to the CNS

### CNS Depressants

- Increased depressive effects of both drugs

### Dronabinol

- Dangerous effect on the CNS

### Muscle Relaxants

- Increased sedation

### Narcotic Analgesics
*Guide 322*

- Increased sedation

### Sedatives

- Increased sedation

### Sleep Inducers

- Increased sedation

### SSRIs *Guide 249*

- Increased sedation

### Tranquilizers

- Increased sedation

## Other Interactions

### Alcohol *Guide 302*

- Increased sedation

### Cocaine *Guide 307*

- Incoordination
- Increased sedation

### Marijuana *Guide 318*

- Incoordination
- Increased sedation
- Drowsiness

## Assessment

- Assess scene safety *Guide 402*
- Use PPE *Guide 002*
- Approach patient *Guide 003*

- Primary and secondary medical survey *Guide 403*
- Medications
- Brief mental status exam *Guide 404*
- Lethality assessment *Guide 407*
- Emotional first aid *Guide 004*

**Reporting**
- Patient description
- Chief complaint
- Medical findings
- Medications and compliance
- Known diagnoses
- Mental status
- Lethality

## (GUIDE 328) ANABOLIC STEROIDS

### Description
- Androgen
- Some prescription uses
- Generic available
- Available as pill, liquid, or skin patch

### Medical Uses
- Augments treatment of aplastic anemia
- Blocks growth of breast cancer cells
- Corrects male hormone deficiencies
- Decreases calcium loss of osteoporosis
- Stimulates growth in dwarfism
- Stimulates onset of puberty in males
- Stimulates weight gain after illness or injury and in chronically underweight individuals

### Generic & Brand Names

*Generic*
- Ethylestrenol
- Fluoxymesterone
- Methyltestosterone
- Nondrolone
- Oxandrolone
- Oxymetholone
- Stanozolol
- Testosterone

*Brand*
- Anabolin
- Anabolin LA
- Anadrol-50
- Anapolon 50
- Andro 100
- Andro-Cyp 100
- Andro-Cyp 200
- Androderm
- Androgel

3

- Android-10
- Android-25
- Android-T
- Andro L.A. 200
- Androlone
- Andronaq-50
- Andronaq-LA
- Andronate 100
- Andronate 200
- Andropository 100
- Andryl 200
- Deca-Durabolin
- Delatest
- Delatestryl
- DepAndro 100
- DepAndro 200
- DepAndrogyn
- Depo-Testadiol
- Depotest
- Depotestogen
- Depo-Testosterone
- Duo-Cyp
- Duo-Gen LA
- Duogex LA
- Dura-Dumone 90/4
- Durabolin
- Durabolin-50
- Duratest-100
- Duratest-200
- Duratestin
- Durathate-200
- Estratest
- Estratest H.S.
- Everone
- Halodrin
- Halotestin
- Histerone-50
- Histerone-100
- Hybolin Decanoate
- Menoject L.A.

- Neo-Pause
- OB
- Premarin with Methytestosterone
- Teev
- Tes Est Cyp
- Test-Estro Cypionate
- Tylosterone
- Valertest No. 1
- Valertest No. 2

## Street Names

- Arnolds
- Gym Candy
- Juice
- Pumpers
- Roids
- Stackers
- Weight Trainers

## Signs & Symptoms

- Hypertension
- Blood clotting
- Acne
- Hair loss
- Increased risk of heart attack
- Increased risk of stroke
- Liver disease
- Kidney disease

### Males

- Testicular shrinkage
- Impotence
- Reduced sperm production
- Increased risk of prostate cancer
- Breast enlargement (gynecomastia)

3

### Females

- Menstrual irregularities
- Decreased breast size
- Deepening of voice
- Facial and body hair
- Clitoral enlargement

### High Doses

- Irritability
- Hostility and aggression
- Difficulty concentrating

### Withdrawal

- Depression *Guide 113*
- Fatigue
- Restlessness
- Loss of appetite
- Insomnia
- Decreased sex drive
- Headache
- Muscle and joint pain
- Body image disorders

## Psychotropic & Other Medication Reactions

### Anticoagulants

- Increased anticoagulant effect

### Antidiabetic agents

- Increased antidiabetic effect

### Insulin

- Increased antidiabetic effect

## Other Interactions

### Salt

- Excessive fluid retention
- Edema

## Assessment

- Assess scene safety *Guide 402*
- Use PPE *Guide 002*
- Approach patient *Guide 003*
- Primary and secondary medical survey *Guide 403*
- Medications
- Brief mental status exam *Guide 404*
- Brief psychosocial history *Guide 405*
- Emotional first aid *Guide 004*

## Reporting

- Patient description
- Chief complaint
- Medical findings
- Medications and compliance
- Mental status

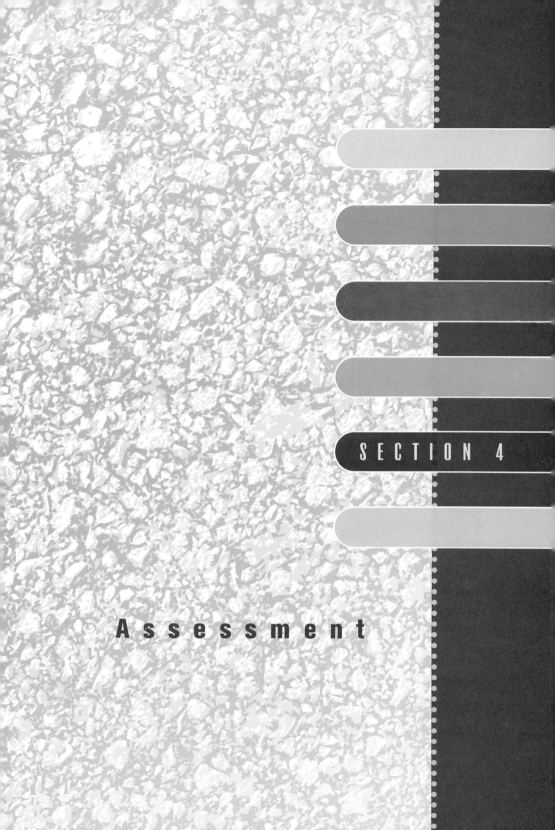

SECTION 4

Assessment

## GUIDE 401 — ASSESSMENT: ALPHABETICAL INDEX

## GUIDE 402 — SCENE SAFETY

### Size Up Potential Hazards

- Animals
- Crime scenes
- Electrical hazards
- Fires
- Glass
- Hazardous materials
- Insects
- Structural instability
- Traffic
- Vehicular damage
- Violence
- Weather

### Body Substance Isolation

- Airborne droplets
- Blood
- Breast Milk
- Cerebrospinal fluid
- Emesis
- Fecal matter or anal secretions
- Oral or nasal secretions
- Respiratory secretions
- Saliva
- Semen
- Tears
- Urine
- Vaginal secretions

### Precautions

- Remove patients from immediate danger
- Use personal protective equipment (PPE) *Guide 002*
- Universal precautions
- Proper disposal of biohazards

**4**

**PRIMARY & SECONDARY MEDICAL ASSESSMENTS**

## Primary Assessment

### Level of Consciousness

- A: Alert
- V: Responsive to voice
- P: Responsive to pain
- U: Unresponsive

### Airway

- Open
- Assess
- Suction
- Secure

### Breathing (Respiration)

- Look
- Listen
- Feel

### Circulation

- Assess for pulse
- Assess for and control obvious bleeding
- Blood pressure
- Capillary refill

### Rapid Trauma Assessment

- Neck
- Chest
- Abdomen
- Pelvis
- Extremities
- Back and buttocks

## Secondary Assessment

### Focused Trauma Assessment

- Assess injuries
- Control bleeding

### Detailed Physical Exam

- Head
- Ears
- Eyes
- Face
- Nose
- Mouth
- Chest
- Abdomen
- Pelvis
- Extremities
- Hands
- Feet
- Back
- Buttocks
- Skin
- Recheck vital signs

### History of Chief Complaint

- Onset
- Provoking factors
- Quality
- Region and radiation
- Severity
- Time/duration
- Interventions and relief

4

*Brief Medical History*

- Symptoms
- Allergies
- Medications

- Pertinent medical history
- Last medical evaluation
- Events preceding call for help

## GUIDE 404 BRIEF MENTAL STATUS EXAM

### Physical Appearance

*Grooming & Hygiene*

- Overall cleanliness
- Hair
- Nails
- Teeth
- Odor

*Clothing*

- Cleanliness
- Neat or disheveled
- Appropriate to weather conditions
- Consistent with social norms
- Atypical or bizarre

*Physical Characteristics*

- Scars
- Tattoos
- Piercings
- Brands
- Amputations
- Deformities
- Disfigurations

### Orientation

- Person
- Place
- Time
- Event

### Posture

- Alert
- Socially appropriate
- Slumped
- Rigid/tense
- Aggressive
- Bizarre

### Facial Expressions

- Socially appropriate
- Anxious, fearful, apprehensive
- Depressed, sad, despondent
- Angry, hostile
- Empty
- Bizarre
- Atypical, inappropriate
- Tics

### Movements & Gestures

- Socially appropriate
- Rapid, accelerated
- Slowed, decreased
- Hostile, aggressive
- Compulsive
- Provocative
- Atypical, peculiar

## Speech

- Eye contact: normal, evasive, fixed
- Volume: unusually loud or soft-spoken
- Rate: socially appropriate, rapid, slow
- Clarity: clear, slurred, stammering, stuttering, mumbling
- Pressured
- Content: socially appropriate, bizarre, delusional, poverty (decreased content)

## Interaction with Evaluator

- Cooperative, uncooperative
- Submissive
- Domineering
- Hostile
- Suspicious
- Seductive
- Distant, distracted

## GUIDE 405 BRIEF PSYCHOSOCIAL HISTORY

### Biographical Information

- Name
- Address
- Phone Number
- Age
- Gender
- Ethnicity
- Relationship status
- Height
- Weight
- Religious preference
- Social Security Number

### Presenting Problem

- Patient's statement of the problem
- Results of primary and secondary medical surveys
- Mental status
- Lethality
- History of the problem: onset, duration, treatment

### Current Medications

- Type: prescription, Over the Counter (OTC), vitamins, supplements
- Prescribed by whom
- Dosage
- Side effects
- Compliance
- Duration of regimen since initiation

### Psychological History

- Psychological disorders
- Date
- Treatment
- Outcome

4

*Current Level of Functioning*

- ADLs (Activities of Daily Living)
- Home life
- Work/school
- Leisure time: interests, hobbies, sports, activities
- Stress management skills

## GUIDE 406 MENTAL STATUS EXAM

### Physical Appearance

*Grooming & Hygiene*

- Overall cleanliness
- Hair
- Nails
- Teeth

*Clothing*

- Cleanliness
- Neat or disheveled
- Appropriate to weather conditions
- Consistent with social norms
- Atypical or bizarre

*Physical Characteristics*

- Scars
- Tattoos
- Piercings
- Brands
- Amputations
- Deformities
- Disfigurations

### Orientation

- Person
- Place
- Time
- Event

### Posture

- Alert
- Socially appropriate
- Slumped
- Rigid/tense
- Aggressive
- Bizarre

### Facial Expressions

- Socially appropriate
- Anxious, fearful, apprehensive
- Depressed, sad, despondent
- Angry, hostile
- Empty
- Bizarre
- Atypical, inappropriate
- Tics

### Movements & Gestures

- Socially appropriate
- Rapid, accelerated
- Slowed, decreased
- Hostile, aggressive
- Compulsive
- Provocative
- Atypical, peculiar

### Speech

- Eye contact: normal, evasive, fixed

- Volume: unusually loud or soft-spoken
- Rate: socially appropriate, rapid, slow
- Clarity: clear, slurred, stammering, stuttering, mumbling
- Pressured
- Content: socially appropriate, bizarre, delusional, poverty (decreased content)

## Interaction with Evaluator

- Cooperative, uncooperative
- Submissive
- Domineering
- Hostile
- Suspicious
- Seductive
- Distant, distracted

## Affect (Mood)

- Socially appropriate to event
- Depressed, sad, despondent
- Flat
- Anxious, fearful, apprehensive
- Angry, hostile
- Blunted
- Euphoric, elated
- Labile (mood swings)
- Bizarre
- Atypical, inappropriate

## Perceptions

- Normal
- Illusions (mistaken perceptions)

## Hallucinations

- Auditory
- Visual
- Tactile
- Olfactory (Smell)
- Gustatory (Taste)

## Cognition (Thought)

### Intellectual Functioning

- Attention: normal, focused, distracted
- Intelligence: normal, bright, gifted, dull, developmentally disabled
- Abstraction: abstract or concrete thought. Use proverbs to test; for example, ask, "What is meant by a rolling stone gathers no moss?"
- Calculation: serial 7's—count backward from 100 by subtracting 7

### Memory

- Recent: describe event
- Short term: What did you have for breakfast?
- Long term: Where were you born?

### Content

- Lethality: suicidal or homicidal
- Delusions: grandeur, paranoid, reference, influence
- Obsessions
- Phobias
- Depersonalization
- Psychotic
- Sociopathic

4

### Associations
- Normal
- Loose
- Bizarre

### Judgment
- Manages ADLs
- Makes reasonable life decisions

- Blames others
- Problem-solving

### Information
- Oriented to time, place, person, and event (oriented × 4)
- Fund of information: president, season, holidays, etc.

## GUIDE 407  LETHALITY ASSESSMENT

### Suicide *Guide 135*

#### Thoughts
- Contemplating suicide
- Wishing to be dead
- Going to sleep and not waking up
- Stop living
- Hopelessness
- Helplessness

#### Intent
- Does the person really want to kill himself or herself?
- Is the person just asking for help?
- Does the person want to get back at someone?
- What problems would suicide solve?

#### Plan
- Does the person have a plan?

- Has the person thought about how to commit suicide?

#### Means
- Does the person have a way to carry out the plan?
- Access to a firearm
- Stockpiling medications
- Other means

### Homicide

#### Thoughts
- Contemplating homicide
- Wishing someone were dead
- Revenge
- Rage and hatred
- Paranoia

#### Intent
- Does the person really want to kill someone?

- Is the person just asking for help?
- Does the person want to get back at someone?
- What problems would homicide solve?

*Plan*

- Does the person have a plan?

- Has the person thought about how to commit homicide?

*Means*

- Does the person have a way to carry out the plan?
- Access to a firearm
- Other weapons
- Other plans

## GUIDE 408 — DETAILED MEDICAL HISTORY

### Biographical Information

- Name
- Address
- Phone number
- Age
- Gender
- Ethnicity
- Relationship status
- Height
- Weight
- Religious preference
- Social Security Number

### Source of History

- Patient
- Family member (specify)
- Friend
- Medical record

### Chief Complaint

- Onset
- Provoking factors
- Description and/or quality
- Radiation
- Region
- Relief
- Severity
- Time/duration

### Present Illnesses/Injuries

- Description/location
- Timing: onset, duration, frequency
- Quality
- Severity or quantity
- Setting in which they occur
- Aggravating factors
- Relieving factors
- Associated manifestations
- Physical disabilities

### Current Medications

- Type: prescription, OTC, vitamins, supplements
- Prescribed by whom
- Dosage
- Side effects
- Compliance

4

- Duration of regimen since initiation
- Home remedies tried

## Allergies
- Medications
- Food
- Contact substances: household products, plants, insects, etc.
- Environmental: pollens, molds, dust, etc.

## Current Health Status
- General health condition as described by the patient
- Ability to perform ADLs
- Sleep patterns
- Diet and nutrition
- Digestion and elimination
- Exercise
- Sexual activity
- Caffeine intake
- Alcohol use
- Tobacco use
- Drug use
- Recent trips to foreign countries
- Social support system

## Health Management
- Primary care physician
- Date of last physical exam
- Routine health screening tests
- Personal hygiene
- Self-examination
- Date of last dental exam
- Date of last vision exam
- Date of last hearing exam
- Personal health goals

## Medical History
### Childhood Illnesses
- Allergies
- Asthma
- Chicken Pox
- Epilepsy
- Measles
- Mumps
- Polio
- Mental illness
- Rheumatic Fever
- Rubella
- Scarlet Fever
- Others
- Treatment and outcomes

### Adult Illnesses
- Anemia
- Alcoholism
- Asthma
- Arthritis
- Bowel problems
- Cancer
- Cholesterol
- Diabetes
- Dizziness
- Endocrine disease
- Headaches
- Heart disease
- Hepatitis
- HIV/AIDS
- Hypertension
- Kidney disease
- Mental illness
- Obesity
- Renal disorders
- Seizures
- Sleep disorders
- Skin disease

4

- Stomach problems
- Stroke
- Tuberculosis
- Others

*Accidents/Injuries*
- Type
- Date
- Treatment
- Outcome

*Hospitalizations*
- Date
- Reason
- Treatment
- Outcome

*Surgeries*
- Type
- Date
- Outcome

*Exposure to Toxins or Environmental Pollutants*
- Type
- Amount of exposure
- Effects

*Blood Transfusions*
- Date
- Number
- Adverse outcomes

*Psychological Treatment*
- Type
- Date
- Treatment
- Outcome

*Obstetric History*
- Number of pregnancies
- Outcomes
- Age at pregnancy
- Type of labor and deliveries
- Complications
- Postpartum condition

*Immunizations: Dates*
- Chicken Pox
- Diphtheria
- Hepatitis
- Influenza
- Measles
- Mumps
- Pertussis (whooping cough)
- Pnuemococcal
- Polio
- Rubella
- Small Pox
- Tetanus

## Family History

*Family Members*
- Age and health of family members: parents, grand-parents, and siblings
- Age and cause of death of family members: parents, grandparents, and siblings
- Age and health of spouse/significant other and children
- Age and cause of death of spouse/significant other and children

4

## Family Medical History

- Alcoholism
- Alzheimer's Disease
- Asthma
- Arthritis
- Cancer
- Diabetes
- Endocrine disease
- Headaches
- Heart disease
- Hepatitis
- HIV/AIDS
- Hypertension
- Kidney disease
- Mental illness
- Obesity
- Renal disorders
- Seizures
- Skin disease
- Stroke
- Tuberculosis
- Other

## GUIDE 409  PSYCHOSOCIAL HISTORY

### Biographical Information

- Name
- Address
- Phone number
- Age
- Gender
- Ethnicity
- Relationship status
- Height
- Weight
- Religious preference
- Social Security Number

### Presenting Problem

- Patient's statement of the problem
- Results of primary and secondary medical surveys
- Mental status
- Lethality
- History of the problem: onset, duration, treatment

### Emotional & Behavioral Assessment

#### Chronological History

- Emotional problems: age of onset, duration, treatment, outcomes
- Behavioral problems: age of onset, duration, treatment, outcomes
- Substance abuse: age of onset, duration, treatment, outcomes

#### Current Level of Functioning

- ADLs
- Home life
- Work/school

- Leisure time: interests, hobbies, sports, activities
- Stress management skills

## Social History

### *Relationship Status*

- Single
- Married
- Significant other
- Divorced
- Widowed

### *Family Status*

- Children: gender and age
- Grandchildren
- Other family members

### *Living Situation*

- Cohabitants: family, roommates, etc.
- Residence: home, apartment, dormitory, and so on

### *Social & Peer Relationships*

- Close friends
- Acquaintances
- Neighbors
- Co-workers
- Others

### *Religious Participation*

- Faith community: church, synagogue, temple, etc.
- Frequency of attendance
- Length of membership

## Drug & Alcohol Use

- Alcohol: types, number of drinks per week
- Tobacco: types, frequency
- Marijuana: frequency
- Other street drugs

## Financial History

- Financial problems
- Bankruptcy
- Public assistance

## Developmental History

- Place of birth
- Planned pregnancy?
- Complications during pregnancy/delivery
- Developmental delays: walking, talking, toileting, dressing, etc.
- Hereditary disorders
- Early health care
- General health during childhood
- Significant illnesses
- Accidents or injuries
- Sleep disturbances: insomnia, nightmares, bedwetting, etc.
- Puberty and sexual development: normal age, early, delayed

## Family History

- Constellation: parents, stepparents, siblings, stepsiblings, etc.
- Family history of presenting problem
- Family history of other emotional/behavioral problems
- Relationship problems

4

- Abuse: physical, sexual, emotional; neglect
- Divorce
- Financial problems
- Substance abuse
- Living situation
- Frequent moves
- Religious participation
- Legal problems

## Emotional & Behavioral History

### Childhood

- Peer relationships
- School problems: academic, peers, truancy
- Deaths and other significant losses
- Runaway
- Drug and alcohol use
- Sexual development: dating, sexual activity
- Suicide attempts
- Delinquency

### Adulthood

- Relationship history
- Family relationships: parents, siblings, etc.
- Peer relations
- Deaths and other significant losses
- Drug and alcohol use

- Criminal behavior
- Suicide attempts
- Sexual history

## Educational History

- Highest grade completed
- Currently in school
- Vocational training
- School difficulties: daydreaming, focusing attention, completing assignments, etc.

## Vocational History

- Current occupation
- Professional licenses and/or certifications
- Length of occupation
- Military service
- Age at retirement
- Chronological history
- Significant periods out of work
- Work habits
- History of employment problems
- Vocational rehabilitation

## Legal History

- Current legal problems: criminal and civil
- History of legal problems: arrests, convictions, etc.
- Civil judgments

4

## Domestic Relationships

- Do you feel that your spouse/partner/family treats you well?
- Does anything happen at home that makes you feel afraid?
- When you have arguments/fights at home, what happens?
- Are you afraid of the consequences of an argument/fight?
- Do you ever change your behavior because you are afraid of those consequences?
- Does your spouse/partner/family break objects in the home during arguments/fights?
- Has your spouse/partner/family ever made you do something that you did not want to do?
- Does your spouse/partner/family criticize you (or your children) all the time?
- Has your spouse/partner/family ever threatened to hurt you (or your children)?
- Has your spouse/partner/family ever put their hands on you (or your children) against your will?
- Has your spouse/partner/family ever hurt your pets?
- Has your spouse/partner/family ever destroyed your (or your children's) clothing, possessions, or other objects that mean a great deal to you?
- Has your spouse/partner/family ever destroyed your home and/or furniture?
- Does your spouse/partner/family abuse drugs or alcohol?
- What happens when they abuse drugs or alcohol?

## Health

- Has your spouse/partner/family ever prevented you from taking medication that you need?
- Has your spouse/partner/family ever prevented you from seeking medical care that you needed?
- Does your spouse/partner/family let you sleep at night?

## Social Relationships

- Does your spouse/partner/family always act jealously?
- Does your spouse/partner/family always call to check up on you?
- Is it hard for you to maintain relationships with your

family, friends, or co-workers because your spouse/partner/family disapproves of them?

- Does your spouse/partner/family ever accuse you unjustly of flirting or having an affair?
- Has your spouse/partner/family ever tried to keep you from leaving the house?
- Does your spouse/partner/family make it hard for you to go to work and/or maintain a job?

## Finances

- Does your spouse/partner/family give you money when you need it?
- Do you know what your family's assets are?
- Do you know where important documents like check books, bank statements, certificates, deeds, and passports are kept?

- If you wanted to look at any of those documents, is it possible for you to do so?
- Does your spouse/partner/family ever spend large sums of money and refuse to tell you what it was spent on?

## Sexual Relationship

- Has your spouse/partner/family ever forced you to have sex?
- Has your spouse/partner/family ever forced you to engage in any type of sexual behavior that you were not comfortable with?
- Does your spouse/partner/family force you to have sex when you are sleeping?
- Does your spouse/partner/family force you to have sex when you are sick?

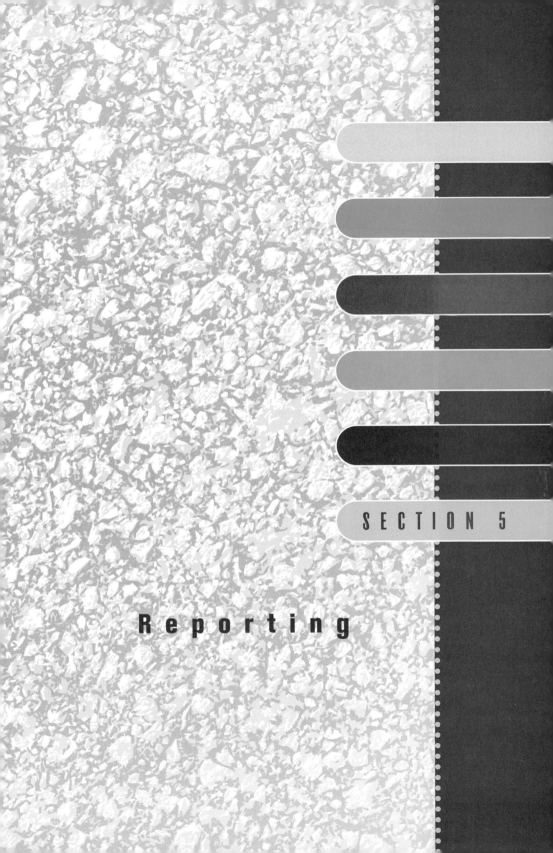

SECTION 5

Reporting

## GUIDE 501 REPORTING: ALPHABETICAL INDEX

## GUIDE 502 ON-SCENE REPORTS

### Information to Include in Initial Radio or Telephone Report

- Unit identification number
- Person providing the report
- Patient's age and gender
- Chief complaint
- Brief history of chief complaint
- Mental status
- Baseline vital signs
- Current medications
- Significant medical history
- Pertinent findings of the primary and secondary medical assessment
- Emergency medical care given
- Response to emergency medical care
- Does medical facility have any questions or orders?
- Unit destination and estimated time of arrival (ETA)

### Information to Report upon Arrival to Hospital Emergency Department

- Patient's age and gender
- Chief complaint
- Brief history of chief compliant
- Mental status *Guide 404*
- Baseline and subsequent vital signs
- Current medications
- Significant medical history
- Pertinent findings of the primary and secondary medical assessments *Guide 403*
- Emergency medical care given
- Response to emergency medical care
- Lethality *Guide 407*
- Detailed medical history *Guide 408*
- Significant psychosocial history *Guide 405*
- Evidence of any abuse

## Physical Abuse

- Battering, beating, injuring, or otherwise physically harming a child under age 18 by a person who is responsible for the child's care and welfare

*May include the following:*

- Beating
- Biting
- Burning
- Hitting
- Kicking
- Pinching
- Pushing
- Shaking
- Shoving
- Striking (with or without an object)

*May also include inappropriate use of the following:*

- Medications
- Medical treatments
- Physical punishment
- Physical restraints

### Signs & Symptoms

- A child's report of being physically abused
- Black eyes
- Bone fractures
- Broken eyeglasses
- Bruises
- Cuts
- Dislocations
- Internal injuries
- Lacerations
- Open wounds
- Punctures
- Rope marks
- Skull fractures
- Sprains
- Untreated injuries at various stages of healing
- Welts

### Behavioral Indicators

- Afraid to go home
- Angry, aggressive, or hyperactive
- Apprehensive when other children cry
- Behavioral extremes
- Frequently absent from or late to school
- Frightened of parents
- Noncommunicative
- Seeks affection from any adult, with no discrimination
- Terrified to make a mess
- Unnaturally dependent
- Wary of adult contacts
- Wears long sleeves or other clothing to hide injuries
- Withdrawn, introverted, passive

### Parental Indicators

- Abuses drugs or alcohol
- Appears anxious or overwhelmed by child's needs

5

- Attempts to conceal child's injury
- Disciplines child too harshly
- Gives different explanations for the same injury
- History of child abuse
- Poor impulse control
- Seems unconcerned about child
- Sees child as bad or evil
- Takes an unusual amount of time to obtain medical care for the child's injury
- Takes child to different doctor or hospital for each injury

## Sexual Abuse

- Any sexual contact
- Coerced nudity
- Forcing or encouraging a child into prostitution
- Sexual assault
- Showing a child pornography
- Taking sexually explicit photographs
- Unwanted touching

### Signs & Symptoms

- A child's report of sexual abuse (children rarely lie about sexual abuse)
- Bruises around the anus, breasts, or genital areas
- Pain or itching in the genital area
- Pregnancy
- Sleep disorders

- Torn, stained, or bloody underclothing
- Unexplained vaginal or anal bleeding
- Venereal disease or genital infection

### Behavioral Indicators

- Bizarre, sophisticated, and/or unusual sexual knowledge or behavior
- Delinquency
- Infantile behavior—sucking, rocking, biting, etc.
- Poor peer relationships
- Refusal to participate in physical education classes
- Running away
- Unusual onset of bed-wetting, nightmares, or thumb-sucking
- Unwilling to change for gym class or other activities
- Wary of adult physical contact
- Withdrawn, introverted, passive

### Parental Indicators

- Abuses drugs or alcohol
- Attempts to conceal child's injury
- Geographically, socially, or emotionally isolated
- History of sexual abuse
- Jealous of child
- Low self-esteem
- Overly protective of child
- Poor impulse control

- Takes an unusual amount of time to obtain medical care for the child's injury
- Takes child to different doctor or hospital for each injury

## Psychological Abuse

- Emotional maltreatment that makes a child feel sad, worthless, and unwanted

*May include the following:*

- Harassment
- Humiliation
- Ignoring
- Insults
- Intimidation
- Isolation from family and friends
- Isolation from preferred activities
- Name-calling
- The "silent treatment"
- Threats
- Verbal assaults

*Signs & Symptoms*

- A child's report of psychological abuse
- Depression
- Failure to thrive
- Sleep disorders
- Speech disorders
- Lags in physical development

*Behavioral Indicators*

- Infantile behavior—sucking, rocking, biting, etc.
- Antisocial or delinquent behavior
- Anger or aggression
- Inhibition of play
- Withdrawn, introverted, passive
- Obsessive Compulsive Disorder *Guide 122*
- Learning disorders
- Attempted suicide *Guide 407*

*Parental Indicators*

- Abuses drugs or alcohol
- Blames or belittles child
- Cold and rejecting
- Demonstrates inconsistent behavior toward child
- Finds nothing good or attractive in the child
- Seems indifferent to child
- Treats children in the family unequally
- Withholds love and affection

## Neglect

- Refusal or failure to provide for a child's physical or emotional needs

*May include the failure or refusal to provide the following:*

- Access to medical and/or dental care
- Adequate supervision
- Clothing
- Comfort
- Food

5

- Medicine
- Personal hygiene
- Personal safety
- Shelter
- Water

*Signs & Symptoms*

- A child's report of neglect
- Consistent hunger
- Poor hygiene
- Inappropriate dress
- Chronically unclean
- Often tired or listless

*Behavioral Indicators*

- Begging or stealing food
- Extended stays in school—early arrival and late departure
- Falling asleep in class
- Frequently absent from or late to school
- Hoarding food
- States there is no caregiver

*Parental Indicators*

- Abuses drugs or alcohol
- Apathetic to life
- Cannot be found
- Chaotic, disorganized home life
- Evidences limited intellectual capability
- Frequently exposes child to unsafe conditions
- History of neglect as a child
- Isolated from family, friends, and neighbors
- Long-term chronic illness
- Seems indifferent to child

## Abandonment

- Abandonment by an individual who has assumed responsibility for providing care
- Abandonment by an individual who has physical custody

*Signs & Symptoms*

- A child's report of being abandoned
- Desertion of a child at a hospital, school, or other institution
- Desertion of a child at a shopping center, supermarket, or other public location

## Assessment

- Assess scene safety *Guide 402*
- Use personal protective equipment (PPE) *Guide 002*
- Primary and secondary medical surveys *Guide 403*
- Medications
- Brief mental status exam *Guide 404*
- Lethality assessment *Guide 407*
- Brief psychosocial history *Guide 405*
- Is this child in imminent danger?
- Is this child in need of emergency services to prevent injury and/or loss?
- What is the nature and extent of the abuse?

5

- Is the abuse likely to occur again?
- What measures are needed to prevent future abuse?

### Reporting

- Description of patient
- Chief complaint
- Medical findings *Guide 403*
- Medications and compliance

- Known diagnoses
- Mental status *Guide 404*
- Lethality *Guide 407*
- Psychosocial history *Guide 405*
- Assessment of abusive situation must be reported to the local child protective services and/or local law enforcement agencies

## GUIDE 504  ELDER ABUSE

### Physical Abuse

- Physical force that may result in bodily injury, physical pain, or impairment

*May include the following:*

- Beating
- Biting
- Burning
- Hitting
- Kicking
- Pinching
- Pushing
- Shaking
- Shoving
- Striking (with or without an object)

*May also include inappropriate use of the following:*

- Force-feeding
- Medications

- Medical treatments
- Physical punishment
- Physical restraints

*Signs & Symptoms*

- An elder's report of being physically abused
- Black eyes
- Bone fractures
- Broken eyeglasses
- Bruises
- Cuts
- Dislocations
- Internal injuries
- Lacerations
- Open wounds
- Punctures
- Rope marks
- Skull fractures
- Sprains
- Untreated injuries at various stages of healing
- Welts

5

## Sexual Abuse

- Coerced nudity
- Nonconsensual sexual contact
- Sexual assault *Guide 133*
- Sexual contact with a person incapable of giving consent
- Showing pornography without consent
- Taking sexually explicit photographs
- Unwanted touching

### Signs & Symptoms

- An elder's report of sexual abuse
- Bruises around the anus, breasts, or genital areas
- Torn, stained, or bloody underclothing
- Unexplained vaginal or anal bleeding
- Unexplained venereal disease or genital infection

## Psychological Abuse

- The infliction of emotional anguish, distress, or pain through verbal and/or non-verbal actions

### May include the following:

- Being treated like a child
- Harassment
- Humiliation
- Ignoring
- Insults
- Intimidation
- Isolation from family and friends
- Isolation from preferred activities
- Name-calling
- The "silent treatment"
- Threats
- Verbal assaults

### Signs & Symptoms

- An elder's report of psychological abuse
- Behavior usually attributed to dementia, i.e., sucking, biting, rocking
- Emotionally upset or agitated
- Noncommunicative
- Socially withdrawn

## Neglect

- Refusal or failure to fulfill any part of obligations or duties to an elder

### May include failure or refusal to provide the following:

- Access to medical and/or dental care
- Clothing
- Comfort
- Food
- Medicine
- Personal hygiene
- Personal safety
- Shelter
- Water

### Signs & Symptoms

- An elder's report of being neglected
- Dehydration
- Hazardous or unsafe living conditions
- Malnutrition
- Poor personal hygiene
- Unattended or untreated health problems
- Unsanitary or unclean living conditions
- Untreated bed sores

## Abandonment

- Abandonment by an individual who has assumed responsibility for providing care
- Abandonment by an individual who has physical custody

### Signs & Symptoms

- An elder's report of being abandoned
- Desertion of an elder at a hospital, nursing facility, or other similar institution
- Desertion of an elder at a shopping center or other public location

## Financial or Material Exploitation

- Improper use of an elder's funds, property, or assets

### May include the following:

- Cashing checks without authorization or permission
- Coercing or deceiving an elder into signing any document
- Forging an elder's signature
- Improper use of conservatorship, guardianship, or power of attorney
- Misusing or stealing money, property, or other assets

### Signs & Symptoms

- An elder's report of financial exploitation
- Discovery of an elder's signature being forged
- Substandard care being provided or bills unpaid despite the availability of adequate funds
- Sudden appearance of previously uninvolved relatives claiming rights to an elder's money and/or property
- Sudden changes in bank account or banking practices
- Sudden changes to wills or other financial documents
- Sudden, unexplained transfers of money to a family member or to someone outside the family
- The inclusion of additional names on an elder's bank signature card
- The provision of services that are not necessary
- Unauthorized use of an ATM card
- Unexplained disappearances of funds or other valuable possessions

5

## Nursing Home–Specific Abuse

- Failure to provide proper care, comfort, and social contact for a patient

### May include the following:
- Failure to communicate with family members
- Inadequate or substandard medical care
- Lack of activity
- Mismanagement of medications
- Poor nutrition
- Poorly trained staff
- Understaffing

### Signs & Symptoms
- An elder's report of being mistreated
- Bed sores
- Dehydration
- Fear of certain staff members
- Frequent "accidents"
- Loss of appetite
- Malnourished
- Rapid weight gain or loss
- Staff not keeping family members informed
- Unusual or unexplained marks on the body
- Plugged or tied off catheters

## Assessment
- Assess scene safety *Guide 402*
- Use PPE *Guide 002*
- Approach patient *Guide 003*

- Primary and secondary medical surveys *Guide 403*
- Medications and compliance
- Brief mental status exam *Guide 404*
- Lethality assessment *Guide 407*
- Brief psychosocial history *Guide 405*
- Is this person in imminent danger?
- Is this person in need of emergency services to prevent injury and/or loss?
- What is the nature and extent of the abuse?
- Is the abuse likely to occur again?
- Is the patient able to make decisions regarding his or her own welfare?
- What measures are needed to prevent future abuse?

## Reporting
- Description of patient
- Chief complaint
- Medical findings *Guide 403*
- Medications and compliance
- Known diagnoses
- Mental status *Guide 404*
- Lethality *Guide 407*
- Psychosocial history *Guide 405*
- Assessment of abusive situation must be reported to the local adult protective services and/or local law enforcement agencies

5

## Dependent Adults

- Disability
- Illness
- Infirmity
- Injury

## Physical Abuse

- Physical force that may result in bodily injury, physical pain, or impairment

*May include the following:*

- Beating
- Biting
- Burning
- Hitting
- Kicking
- Pinching
- Pushing
- Shaking
- Shoving
- Striking (with or without an object)

*May also include inappropriate use of the following:*

- Force-feeding
- Medications
- Medical treatments
- Physical punishment
- Physical restraints

## Signs & Symptoms

- A dependent adult's report of being physically abused
- Black eyes
- Bone fractures
- Broken eyeglasses
- Bruises
- Cuts
- Dislocations
- Internal injuries
- Lacerations
- Open wounds
- Punctures
- Rope marks
- Skull fractures
- Sprains
- Untreated injuries at various stages of healing
- Welts
- Plugged or tied off catheters

## Sexual Abuse

- Coerced nudity
- Nonconsensual sexual contact
- Sexual assault *Guide 133*
- Sexual contact with a person incapable of giving consent
- Showing pornography without consent
- Taking sexually explicit photographs
- Unwanted touching

5

### Signs & Symptoms

- A dependent adult's report of sexual abuse
- Bruises around the anus, breasts, or genital areas
- Torn, stained, or bloody underclothing
- Pregnancy
- Unexplained vaginal or anal bleeding
- Unexplained venereal disease or genital infection

## Psychological Abuse

- The infliction of emotional anguish, distress, or pain through verbal and/or non-verbal actions

### May include the following:

- Being treated like a child
- Harassment
- Humiliation
- Ignoring
- Insults
- Intimidation
- Isolation from family and friends
- Isolation from preferred activities
- Name-calling
- The "silent treatment"
- Threats
- Verbal assaults

### Signs & Symptoms

- A dependent adult's report of psychological abuse

- Behavior usually attributed to dementia, i.e., sucking, biting, rocking
- Emotionally upset or agitated
- Noncommunicative
- Socially withdrawn

## Neglect

- Refusal or failure to fulfill any part of obligations or duties to an elder

### May include failure or refusal to provide the following:

- Access to medical and/or dental care
- Clothing
- Comfort
- Food
- Medicine
- Personal hygiene
- Personal safety
- Shelter
- Water

### Signs & Symptoms

- A dependent adult's report of being neglected
- Dehydration
- Hazardous or unsafe living conditions
- Malnutrition
- Poor personal hygiene
- Unattended or untreated health problems
- Unsanitary or unclean living conditions
- Untreated bed sores

## Abandonment

- Abandonment by an individual who has assumed responsibility for providing care
- Abandonment by an individual who has physical custody

### Signs & Symptoms

- A dependent adult's report of being abandoned
- Desertion of a dependent adult at a hospital, nursing facility, or other similar institution
- Desertion of a dependent adult at a shopping center or other public location

## Financial or Material Exploitation

- Improper use of a dependent adult's funds, property, or assets

### May include the following:

- Cashing checks without authorization or permission
- Coercing or deceiving a dependent adult into signing any document
- Forging a dependent adult's signature
- Improper use of conservatorship, guardianship, or power of attorney
- Misusing or stealing money, property, or other assets

### Signs & Symptoms

- A dependent adult's report of financial exploitation
- Discovery of a dependent adult's signature being forged
- Substandard care being provided or bills left unpaid despite the availability of adequate funds
- Sudden appearance of previously uninvolved relatives claiming rights to a dependent adult's money and/or property
- Sudden changes in bank account or banking practices
- Sudden changes to financial documents
- Sudden, unexplained transfers of money to a family member or to someone outside the family
- The inclusion of additional names on a dependent adult's bank signature card
- The provision of services that are not necessary
- Unauthorized use of an ATM card
- Unexplained disappearances of funds or other valuable possessions

## Nursing Home–Specific Abuse

- Failure to provide proper care, comfort, and social contact for a patient

5

### May include the following:
- Failure to communicate with family members
- Inadequate or substandard medical care
- Lack of activity
- Mismanagement of medications
- Poor nutrition
- Poorly trained staff
- Understaffing

### Signs & Symptoms
- A dependent adult's report of being mistreated
- Bed sores
- Dehydration
- Fear of certain staff members
- Frequent "accidents"
- Loss of appetite
- Malnourished
- Rapid weight gain or loss
- Staff not keeping family members informed
- Unusual or unexplained marks on the body

### Assessment
- Assess scene safety *Guide 402*
- Use PPE *Guide 002*
- Approach patient *Guide 003*
- Primary and secondary medical surveys *Guide 403*
- Medications

- Brief mental status exam *Guide 404*
- Lethality assessment *Guide 407*
- Brief psychosocial history *Guide 405*
- Is this person in imminent danger?
- Is this person in need of emergency services to prevent injury and/or loss?
- What is the nature and extent of the abuse?
- Is the abuse likely to occur again?
- Is this person able to make decisions regarding his or her own welfare?
- What measures are needed to prevent future abuse?

### Reporting
- Description of patient
- Chief complaint
- Medical findings *Guide 403*
- Medications and compliance
- Known diagnoses
- Mental status *Guide 404*
- Lethality *Guide 407*
- Psychosocial history *Guide 405*
- Assessment of abusive situation must be reported to the local adult protective services and/or local law enforcement agencies

**Activities of daily living (ADL):** Used to describe a person's level of functioning via his/her ability to perform tasks that are considered to be a part of a daily routine such as bathing, feeding oneself, going to work, playing etc.

**Adolescence:** The period of development marked at the beginning by the onset of puberty and at the end by the attainment of physiological or psychological maturity.

**Adolescent onset:** Maladies in which the onset is usually during the adolescent years.

**Agitation:** A state of mental and/or physical restlessness.

**Agnosia:** A state in which objects can be recognized but the person is unable to consciously recognize and interpret their meaning.

**ALOC:** An acronym describing a patient who did not experience a loss of consciousness.

**Alogia:** Occasionally a synonym for aphasia. A condition marked by speech that is dramatically reduced in amount or content (or both). Often described as a poverty of speech.

**Amensia:** Any partial or complete loss of memory. A number of specific forms of amnesia are recognized, each denoting a particular kind of deficit in memory.

**Angina pectoris:** A disease of the heart caused by insufficient blood/oxygen supply and is manifested by intermittent attacks of severe chest pain with a sense of suffocating pressure.

**Antiemetics:** A group of drugs used to treat nausea and vomiting.

**Anxiety:** A vague, unpleasant emotional state with qualities of apprehension, dread, distress, and uneasiness.

**Amenorrhea:** Absence of three or more consecutive menstrual cycles without pregnancy.

**Aphasia:** A general term covering any partial or complete loss of language abilities. The origins are always organic. There are literally dozens of varieties of aphasia.

**Apraxia:** From the Greek, meaning without action. Partial or complete loss of the ability to perform purposive movements.

**Ataxia:** Partial or complete loss of coordination of voluntary muscular movements.

**Autonomic hyperactivity:** Accelerated heart rate, hypertension, and increased respirations.

**Avolition:** Lacking in initiative; the inability to start and persist in goal-directed activity.

**Blunted affect:** A disturbance in affect characterized by sharply reduced intensity of emotional expression.

**Bradycardia:** Abnormally slow heart beat.

**Capillary refill:** The rate in which the minute blood vessels in the fingers and toes refill with blood after a brief occlusion.

**Cardiac arrhythmias:** Heart rhythms that are other than what would be considered normal.

**Cataplexy:** A sudden loss of muscle tone resulting in the individual collapsing "like a sack of potatoes". It may result from a sudden emotional shock or a stroke and is an occasional symptom in narcolepsy.

**Catatonic behavior:** The presence of catatonia as manifested by motoric immobility, excessive motor activity (that is apparently purposeless and not influenced by external stimuli), extreme negativism or mutism, peculiarities of voluntary movement, or echolalia or echopraxia.

**Central nervous system (CNS):** That component of the nervous system composed of the brain, the spinal cord, and their associated neural processes.

**Child onset:** Physical or psychological maladies characterized by their frequent onset in the years of childhood (typically birth and puberty).

**CNS stimulant:** Drugs, including narcotics, when introduced to the body serve to directly stimulate the Central Nervous System.

**Cognition:** A broad (almost unspecifiably so) term that has been traditionally used to refer to such activities as thinking, conceiving, reasoning, etc. Most psychologists use it to refer to any class of mental "behaviors" where the underlying characteristics are of an abstract nature and involve symbolizing, insight, expectancy, complex rule use, imagery, belief, intentionality, and problem solving.

**Cognitive deficits:** (see cognition) The temporary or permanent inability to perform cognitive functions such as symbolizing, insight, expectancy, complex rule use, imagery, belief, intentionality, problem-solving, and other cognitive functions. May be caused by disease, medication, brain injury, drug abuse, or medication.

**Cognitive functions:** (see cognition) The ability to think abstractly, use symbols, utilize complex rules, possess insight, etc.

**Coma:** The abnormal state of deep stupor with total absence of consciousness, loss of all voluntary behavior and most reflexes. The term is reserved for cases resulting from injury, disease, or other trauma.

**Compulsions:** Behavior motivated by factors that compel a person to act against his or her own wishes (also see impulse and obsession).

**Confabulation:** Making up details or filling in the gaps in memory. There may be a conscious act in which one is adding to elaborating partial memories of events or an unconscious act in which falsification serves as a defense mechanism.

**Conjunctiva:** Mucous membranes that line the eyelid and corners of the eyeball.

**Conjunctival injection:** Red/bloodshot eyes.

**Convulsion:** A sudden, violent, extensive seizure with involuntary muscular contraction and relaxation.

**Coprolalia:** Complex vocal tic involving the excessive utterance of obscenities.

**Delirium:** Disturbance of consciousness and cognition.

**Delirium tremors:** Tremors usually caused by alcohol withdrawal.

**Delusions:** A belief that is maintained in spite of argument, data, and refutation, which should be (reasonably) sufficient to destroy it. Care should be taken in the use of the term—one person's delusion may be another's salvation.

**Delusions of grandeur:** A delusional disorder that typically takes the form of believing that one has some great but unrecognized talent or insight.

**Delusions of influence:** Delusional state in which one feels he or she has a special power or ability to directly influence the behavior of others beyond that which would be considered normal influence.

**Delusions of reference:** Delusion in which one interprets remarks or references that are neutral or intended for others as having negative significance for oneself.

**Depersonalization:** In psychiatric terms, it represents an emotional disorder in which there is a loss of contact with one's own personal reality, a strangeness and an unreality of experience. In severe cases, parts of one's body feel alien or altered in size and one may have the experience of perceiving oneself from a distance.

**Detachment:** Generally, a sense of emotional freedom, the lack of feeling of emotional involvement in a problem, with a situation, other person, etc.

**Developmentally disabled:** A general term for any significant handicap appearing in childhood or early adolescence (the criterion often stated is prior to age 18) and which will continue for the life of the individual.

**Diuretic:** Any substance that causes increased secretion and passage of urine.

**Dysarthria:** A general term used in describing defective speech or impaired articulation.

**Dyskinesia:** Deficits in voluntary movement.

**Dysphoric mood:** Depressed mood.

**Dystonia:** Muscular weakness.

**Echolalia:** The compulsive, senseless repetition of a word or phrase just spoken by another.

**Echopraxia:** Pathological tendency to repeat the gestures made by others.

**Edema:** The collection of excess fluid in a part of the body (e.g. pedal edema, pulmonary edema, etc.).

**Euphoria:** A sense of extreme elation generally accompanied by optimism and a deep sense of well-being and heightened activity. In pathological cases it may be totally unrealistic, contain delusions of grandeur and invulnerability and include manic levels of activity.

**Flat affect:** The absence of appropriate, outward emotional responses.

**Grand mal seizure:** Type of severe seizure associated with epilepsy and characterized by two distinct types of seizure activity; decorticate (extremities toward the body core) and deceberate (extremities away from the body core).

**Grandiosity:** The state of feeling that one has some great but unrecognized talent or insight.

**Gustatory:** The sense of taste.

**Gynecomastia:** The development of breasts on a male. The condition may occur spontaneously, through hormone malfunction, or as a direct result of hormone treatments.

**Hallucinations:** A perceptual experience with all the compelling subjective properties of a real sensory impression but without the normal physical stimulus for that sensory modality. Hallucinations are taken as classic indicators of a psychotic disturbance and are a hallmark of various disorders like schizophrenia. In actual usage the term is generally modified so that the particular modality involved is specified; auditory, tactile, visual.

**Huntington's chorea:** Neurological disorder marked by muscular twitching and jerky, involuntary movement.

**Hyperactivity:** Vigorous, inappropriate motor activity.

**Hyperacusis:** Painful sensitivity to sounds, excellent hearing.

**Hyperglycemia:** Increased blood sugar.

**Hypersomnia:** A sleep disorder characterized by excessive sleeping, uncontrollable sleepiness.

**Hypertension:** A condition marked by abnormally elevated blood pressure.

**Hyperthymia:** Excessive emotionality, excitability.

**Hypervigilance:** State of being associated with extreme carefulness, awareness to the possibility of danger or injury.

**Hypoglycemia:** Decreased blood sugar.

**Hypotension:** A condition marked by abnormally low blood pressure.

**Impulse:** This term has a variety of uses, all of which revolve around the core meaning: Any act or event "triggered" by a stimulus and occurring with short latency and with little or no conscious control or direction.

**Impulsivity:** The tendency to act impulsively.

**Incoordination:** State of being uncoordinated in speech, physical movement, or thought.

**Infantile Autisim:** A rare but seriously pathological syndrome, appearing in childhood, characterized by a withdrawn state, a lack of social responsiveness or interest in others, serious communicative and linguistic impairments, and a failure to develop normal attachments, all frequently accompanied by a variety of bizarre ways of responding to the environment, usually including a fascination with inanimate objects and an insistence on routine, order, and sameness.

**Insomnia:** A general term for chronic inability to sleep normally, as evidenced by difficulty in falling asleep, frequent waking during the night, and/or early morning waking with attendant difficulty falling back to sleep. Usually caused by anxiety or pain.

**Intellectual functioning:** The ability to function within normal expectation.

**Lethality:** A term used to describe just how serious a person's determination to commit suicide is.

**Lethality assessment:** A psychological test conducted in an effort to determine a person's determination to commit suicide.

**Lethargy:** Extreme lack of energy or vitality.

**Libido:** Emotional energy or urge, especially that associated with sexual desire.

**Loss of consciousness (LOC):** A medical acronym used in reporting that a patient has experienced or is experiencing a loss of consciousness.

**Maladaptive behavior:** Patterns of behavior likely to produce so much psychic distress that therapy is needed.

**Manic depression:** The phase of a depressive episode manifesting itself via euphoric behavior, extreme happiness, hyperactivity, and feelings of invincibility.

**Mental status:** The level of an individual's mental functioning.

**Mental status exam:** A full clinical work-up of a psychiatric patient including assessment of overall psychiatric condition, diagnosis of existing disorders, prognosis, estimates of suitability for treatment of various kinds, formulation of overall personality, compilation of historical and developmental data, etc.

**Migraine headache:** A severe debilitating headache.

**Mood stabilizer:** An umbrella term for several classes of drugs that are used in the treatment of major mood disorders. All function to stabilize the patient's affect. Included are the tricyclic compounds and the monoamine oxidase (MAO) inhibitors, both of which are used for depression, and lithium, which is used for bipolar disorders.

**Narcolepsy:** An organic sleep disorder characterized by recurrent, uncontrollable, brief episodes of sleep.

**Narcotic:** In psychopharmacology, any drug that has both sedative and analgesic properties. Hence, the classification is restricted to the opiates and opiate-like drugs.

**Narcotic antagonist:** Any drug that functions as a narcotic antagonist. Included are naloxone, methadone, and other agents that are structurally similar to the opiates and presumably function by competing with them for the receptor sites in the central nervous system.

**Neurological:** Having to do with the central nervous system.

**Nystagmus:** Jerky eye movements—vertical or horizontal.

**Obsession:** Any idea that haunts, hovers, and constantly invades one's consciousness. Obsessions are seemingly beyond one's "will" and awareness of their inappropriateness is of little or no avail.

**Olfactory:** The sense of, or act of, smelling.

**Oriented Times Four:** A series of questions utilized in an effort to determine a patient's level consciousness. The knowledge of date, place, time, and event are often utilized to formulate this determination.

**Osteoporosis:** A degenerative disease of the bones usually associated with aging and most frequently found in females.

**OTC:** Over The Counter—an acronym used to describe drugs and medications that can be legally purchased without a prescription.

**Panic Attack:** A discrete period of intense fear or discomfort accompanied by various symptoms that may include shortness of breath, dizziness, palpitations, trembling, sweating, nausea, and often a fear that one is going crazy. The attacks are initially unexpected and typically last no longer than 15 minutes.

**Pellagra:** A disease that occurs when a person does not get enough niacin. It is characterized by scaly skin, sores, diarrhea, inflamed mucous membranes, and mental confusion and delusions. It may develop after gastrointestinal diseases or alcoholism.

**Perceptual disturbances:** A disturbance of those processes that give coherence and unity to sensory input.

**Petit mal seizure:** A mild seizure, usually without loss of consciousness, associated with a mild form of epilepsy.

**Psychological disorder:** Disorders associated with the mind, psyche, and the behaviors manifested by the disorder.

**Psychological history:** An individual's entire mental health history.

**Psychomotor agitation:** Excessive motor activity that is marked by nonproductivity and repetitiveness and associated with feelings of inner tension. Typical behaviors are an inability to remain seated, constant pacing, hand-wringing, tugging and fussing with one's clothes, and rapid, complaining speech.

**Psychomotor retardation:** A general slowing down of motor action, movements, and speech. Seen as a common symptom of various disorders, notably depression.

**Psychosis:** Originally, but now rarely, the total mental condition of a person at a specific moment.

**Psychosocial history:** The systematic gathering of an individual's mental and social functioning.

**Psychotic:** Pertaining to a psychotic disorder. Often used in combined form to mark a disorder when the symptoms are characteristic of or strongly resemble a psychosis.

**Serotonin:** A neurotransmitter found in neural pathways of peripheral ganglia and in the central nervous system. It is an inhibitory transmitter whose actions have been implicated in various processes including sleep, pain, and the psychobiology of various affective disorders, specifically depression and bipolar disorder.

**Stupor:** A general condition characterized by extreme unresponsiveness, lethargy, and loss of orientation.

**Sublingual:** Under the tongue. Usually associated with medications that are placed under the tongue, resulting in fast activation.

**Synergistic:** The combined effect of drugs, etc., that exceeds the sum of their individual effects.

**Tachycardia:** Rapid heart beat.

**Vasoconstrictor:** Any drug or medication that serves to restrict circulation in the vascular system.

**Voluntary posturing:** Voluntary assumptions of inappropriate or bizarre positions.

American Psychiatric Association. (1994). *Diagnostic and Statistical Manual of Mental Health Disorders*, 4th ed. Washington, DC: American Psychiatric Association.

Assad, G. (1995). *Understanding Mental Disorders Due to Medical Conditions or Substance Abuse*. New York, NY: Brunner/Mazel Publishers.

Asken, M. J. (1993). *PsycheResponse: Psychological Skills for Optimal Performance by Emergency Responders*. Englewood Cliffs, NY: Brady.

Bates, B. (1995). *A Guide to Physical Examination and History Taking*, 2nd ed. Philadelphia, PA: J. B. Lippincott Company.

Betts, T., & Kenwood, C. (1992). *Practical Psychiatry*. New York, NY: Oxford University Press.

Brunacini, A. V. (1996). *Essentials of Fire Department Customer Service*. Stillwater, OK: Fire Protection Publications.

Cade, B., & O'Hanlon, W. H. (1993). *A Brief Guide to Brief Therapy*. New York, NY: W. W. Norton & Company.

Cantelme, P. (1995). *Phoenix Firefighters' Customer Service Guide*. Phoenix, AZ: Phoenix Fire Department Production Team.

Caplan, G., & Caplan, R. B. (1993). *Mental Health Consultation and Collaboration*. San Francisco, CA: Jossey-Bass.

Carlson, N. R. (1995). *Foundations of Physiological Psychology*, 3rd ed. Boston, MA: Allyn & Bacon.

Coon, D. (1980). *Introduction to Psychology*, 5th ed. St. Paul, MN: West Publishing Company.

Corey, G., Corey, M. S., & Callahan, P. (1993). *Issues and Ethics in the Helping Professions*, 4th ed. Belmont, CA: Brooks/Cole Publishing Company.

Elling, B., & Elling, K. M. (2002). *The Paramedic Review*. Albany, NY: Delmar Thomson Learning.

Elling, B., & Elling, K. M. (2003). *Principles of Patient Assessment in EMS*. Albany, NY: Delmar Thomson Learning.

Elling B., Elling K. M., & Rothenberg, M. A. (2002). *Why-Driven EMS Enrichment*. Albany, NY: Delmar Thomson Learning.

*Emergency Response Guidebook.* (2000). Washington, DC: US Department of Transportation Research and Special Programs, Administration Office of Hazardous Materials Initiatives and Training.

Emery, G., & Campbell, J. (1986). *Rapid Relief from Emotional Distress.* New York, NY: Ballantine Books.

Evers, D. Miller, M., & Glover, T. (2003). *Pocket Partner for Law Enforcement.* Littleton, CO: Sequoia Publishing, Inc.

*Firefighter's Safety/Survival Guide.* (1996). Phoenix, AZ: Corporate Communications, Publications Section.

Gregory, R. J. (1992). *Psychological Testing: History, Principles, and Applications.* Boston, MA: Allyn & Bacon.

Hafen, B. Q., & Frandsen, K. J. (1985). *Psychological Emergencies & Crisis Intervention.* Englewood Cliffs, NJ: Prentice Hall.

Jacobs, D. T. (1991). *Patient Communication for First Responders and EMS Personnel.* Englewood Cliffs, NJ: Brady.

Kaplan, H. I., & Sadock, B. J. (1993). *Pocket Handbook of Psychiatric Drug Treatment.* Baltimore, MD: Williams & Wilkins.

Kastenbaum, R. J. (1991). *Death, Society and Human Experience*, 5th ed. Boston, MA: Allyn & Bacon.

Kazdin, A. E. (1989). *Behavior Modification in Applied Settings*, 4th ed. Pacific Grove, CA: Brooks/Cole Publishing Company.

Konopasek, D. E. (2003). *Medication Fact Sheets: A Behavioral Medication Reference Guide for the Education Professional.* Longmont, CO: Sopris West Educational Services.

Kubler-Ross, E. (1981). *Living with Death and Dying.* New York, NY: Macmillan Publishing Company.

Kubler-Ross, E. (1969). *On Death and Dying: What the Dying have to Teach Doctors, Nurses, Clergy and their Own Families.* New York, NY: Macmillan Publishing Company.

Leasia, M. S., & Monahan, F. D. (2002). *A Practical Guide to Health Assessment*, 2nd ed. Philadelphia, PA: W. B. Saunders Company.

Matheny, K. B. (1992). *Stress and Strategies for Lifestyle Management.* Atlanta, GA: Georgia State University Business Press.

Maxmen, J. S., & Ward, N. G. (1995). *Psychotropic Drugs: Fast Facts*, 2nd ed. New York, NY: W. W. Norton Company.

Millon, T., & Everly, G. S. (1985). *Personality and Its Disorders: A Biosocial Approach.* New York, NY: John Wiley & Sons.

Mitchell, J., & Bray, G. (1990). *Emergency Services Stress.* Englewood Cliffs, NJ: Brady.

Reber, A. S. (1995). *Dictionary of Psychology*, 2nd ed. New York, NY: Penguin Books, Ltd.

Rothman, J. (1994). *Practice with Highly Vulnerable Clients: Case Management and Community-Based Service.* Englewood Cliffs, NJ: Prentice Hall.

Russo, R. J. (1980). *Serving and Surviving as a Human-Service Worker.* Prospect Heights, IL: Waveland Press.

Soreff, S. M., & Cadigan, R. T. (2003). *EMS Street Strategies: Effective Patient Interaction*, 2nd ed. Clifton Park, NY: Delmar Learning.

Talmon, M. (1990). *Single Session Therapy: Maximizing the Effect of the First (and Often Only) Therapeutic Encounter*. San Francisco, CA: Jossey-Bass.

Thio, M. (1990). *Deviant Behavior*, 4th ed. New York, NY: HarperCollins College.

Thompson, J. M., & Bowers, A. C. (1992). *Health Assessment: An Illustrated Pocket Guide*. St. Louis, MO: Mosby Year-Book.

Townsend, M. C. (2001). *Nursing Diagnoses in Psychiatric Nursing: Care Plans and Psychotropic Medications*, 5th ed. Philadelphia, PA: F. A. Davis Company.

Urbaitis, J. C. (1983). *Psychiatric Emergencies*. Norwalk, CT: Appleton-Century-Crofts.

Vacc, N. A., Wittmer, J., & Devaney, S. (1988). *Experiencing and Counseling Multicultural and Diverse Populations*, 2nd ed. Muncie, IN: Accelerated Development.

Watson, D. L. (1993). *Self-Directed Behavior: Self-Modification for Personal Adjustment*, 6th ed. Pacific Grove, CA: Brooks/Cole Publishing Company.

Weber, J. (1993). *Nurses' Handbook of Health Assessment*, 2nd ed. Philadelphia, PA: J. B. Lippincott Company.

Weiten, W., & Lloyd, M. A. (1994). *Psychology Applied to Modern Life*. Pacific Grove, CA: Brooks/Cole Publishing Company.

Zastrow, C. (1993). *Social Work with Groups*, 3rd ed. Chicago, IL: Nelson-Hall Publishers.

Calmylin with Codeine, 179
Cancer, marijuana for, 196–199
Candy, 173, 177
Capillary refill, 250
Captain Cody, 180
Carbamazepine, 99–100
    for alcohol abuse, 165
    for bipolar disorder, 16
    for conduct disorder, 17
    for paranoia, 39
    for schizophrenia, 48
Carbex, 135
Carbidopa and levodopa, 41,
        100–101
Carbolith, 114
Cardiac arrhythmias
    beta-blockers for, 93–95
    definition of, 250
Carisoprodol, 212
Carteolol, 93
Cartrol, 94
Carvedilol, 93
Cataplexy, 250
Catapres, 103
Catapres-TTS, 103
Catatonic behavior, 250
Catatonic schizophrenia, 48
Cat Valiums, 194–195
Celexa, 136
Central nervous system
        (CNS), 250
Central nervous system (CNS)
        stimulant, 250
Centrax, 91, 173
Chalk, 168
Charlie, 177
Cheracol, 179
Child abuse, 237–241
Child onset, 250
Children, suicide in, 53, 54
China Girl, 185
China White, 185
Chloral hydrate, 101–102, 175–176
Chlordiazepoxide, 91, 172
Chlorgest-HD, 204
Chlorpromanyl-5, 132
Chlorpromanyl-20, 132
Chlorpromanyl-40, 132

Chlorpromazine, 131
Cholinesterase inhibitors,
        102–103
    for Alzheimer's, 12
    for dementia, 23
Christmas, 175
Christmas Rolls, 175
Chronic, 196
Cibalith-S, 114
Cirrhosis, thiamine for, 137–138
Citalopram, 136
Citra Forte, 204
Clarity, 184
Cleaning fluids, 193–194
Clindex, 91, 173
Clinoxide, 91, 173
Clomipramine, 82
Clonazepam, 91, 172
Clonidine, 103–104
Clorazepate, 91, 172
Clozapine, 104–105
    for conduct disorder, 17
    for paranoia, 39
    for schizophrenia, 48
    for Tourette's disorder, 55
Clozaril, 104
CNS. *See* Central nervous system
CoActifed, 179
CoActifed Expectorant, 179
Cocaine, 176–178
    withdrawal, tricyclics for, 83
Codehist DH, 179
Codeine, 179–182
Codeine sulfate, 179
Codeine and terpin hydrate, 179
Codiclear DH, 204
Codimal DH, 204
Codimal PH, 179
Cody, 180
Cogentin, 84
Co-Gesic, 204
Cognex, 102
    for Alzheimer's, 12
    for dementia, 23
Cognition, 250
Cognitive deficits, 250
Cognitive functions, 250–251
Coke, 177

Dolmar, 89, 170
Domestic violence, 27–28, 233–234
Donepezil, 102
Doors and Fours, 180
Dopar, 113
Dope, 191, 197
Doral, 91, 173
Dormarex 2, 85
Dormin, 85
Doxepin, 82
Drixoral, 183
Drug and alcohol abuse, assessment of, 229
Drugs of abuse, 146–164. *See also specific drugs*
D's Dance, 212
Duocet, 204
Duo-Cyp, 216
Duo-Gen L.A., 216
Duogex LA, 216
Duo-Medihaler, 132
Durabolin, 216
Durabolin-50, 216
Dura-Dumone 90/4, 216
Duragesic, 185
Duralith, 114
Duramorph, 200
Duratest-100, 216
Duratest-200, 216
Duratestin, 216
Durathate 200, 216
Dwarfism, anabolic steroids for, 215–217
DX, 183
Dysarthria, 252
Dyskinesia, 252
Dysphoric mood, 252
Dystonia, 252

E
Eating disorders, 28–30
Echolalia, 252
Echopraxia, 252
Ecstasy, 184–185
Edema
    beta-blockers for, 93–95

definition of, 252
Educational history, 232
Effexor, 143
    for anxiety disorder, 15
    for depression, 25
    for dissociative identity disorder, 26
    for phobias, 46
    for post-traumatic stress disorder, 47
Effexor XR, 143
Elavil, 82
Elavil Plus, 82, 132
Eldepryl, 135
Elderly
    abuse of, reporting, 241–244
    suicide in, 54
Embalming Fluid, 209
Emergencies, 8–9. *See also specific emergencies*
Emotional and behavioral history, 232
Emotional assessment, 230–231
Endep, 82
Endocet, 204
Endolor, 89, 170
Endur-Acin, 127
Epilepsy
    barbiturates for, 90–91, 170–172
    divalproex for, 106–107
    valproic acid for, 141–142
Epimorph, 200
Epitol, 99
Epival, 106
Equanil, 120
Equanil Wyseals, 120
Ergoloid mesylates, 107–108
    for dementia, 23
    for depression, 24
Ergotamine, belladonna, and phenobarbital, 14, 108–109
Escitalopram, 136
Esgic, 89, 170
Esgic-Plus 4, 89, 170
Eskalith, 114
Eskalith CR, 114

for conduct disorder, 17–18
for obsessive-compulsive
    disorder, 36
for personality disorders, 42
Lithobid, 114
Lithonate, 114
Lithotabs, 114
Litizine, 114
Loads, 180
Locker Room, 194
Loftran, 92, 173
Lopressor, 94
Lopressor SR, 94
Lorazepam, 91, 172
Lorazepam Intensol, 92, 173
Lorcet, 204
Lortab, 204
Loss of consciousness (LOC), 253
Love Boat, 209
Love pills, 184
Loxapac, 115
Loxapine, 115–116
    for anxiety disorder, 14
    for depression, 24
    for dissociative identity
        disorder, 26
    for phobias, 46
    for schizophrenia, 49
Loxitane, 115
Loxitane C, 115
LSD. *See* Lysergic acid
    diethylamide
Ludiomil, 118
    for depression, 24
    for dissociative identity
        disorder, 26
Luminal, 90, 171
Lysergic acid diethylamide
    (LSD), 51, 195–196

M
M, 200
Magic Mushrooms, 203
Majeptil, 132
Maladaptive behavior, 253
Male hormone deficiencies,
    anabolic steroids for,
    215–217

Mallergan-VC with Codeine, 179
Mania, 15
    olanzapine for, 128
Manic depression, 253
MAOIs. *See* Monoamine oxidase
    inhibitors
Maprotiline, 118
    for depression, 24
    for dissociative identity
        disorder, 26
Marax, 112
Marax DF, 112
Marflex, 128
Marijuana, 196–199
Marnal, 90, 171
Mazepine, 99
MDMA, 184–185
Mebaral, 171, 90
Medical history, 227–230
Medigesic, 90, 171
Medilium, 92, 173
Medi-Tran, 120
Mellaril, 132
Mellaril Concentrate, 132
Mellaril-S, 132
Menoject-LA, 216
Mental status, 253
Mental status exam, 224–226
    brief, 222–223
    definition of, 253–254
Meperidine and acetaminophen,
    204
Mephobarbital, 89, 170
Meprobamate, 119–120
    for anxiety disorder, 14
    for dissociative identity
        disorder, 26
Meprospan 200, 120
Meprospan 400, 120
Mesc, 199
Mescal, 199
Mescaline, 199
Mesoridazine, 131
Metadate
    for attention deficit
        disorders, 11
    for depression, 24
    for narcolepsy, 35

Metadate CD, 121, 210
Metadate ER, 121, 210
Meth, 168
Methamphetamine, 80, 168
Metharbital, 89, 170
Methotrimeprazine, 131
3-4 Methylenedioxymethamphet-
    amine, 184–185
Methylin ER, 121, 210
Methylphenidate, 121–122, 210
    for attention deficit
        disorders, 11
    for depression, 24
    for narcolepsy, 35
Methyltestosterone, 215
Metoprolol, 94
Meval, 92, 173
Mexican Valium, 212
Mickey Finn, 175
Micro, 195
Microdot, 195
Midahist DH, 179
Midazolam, 91, 172
Migraine headaches
    clonidine for, 103–104
    definition of, 254
    divalproex for, 106–107
    MAOIs for, 116–118
Miltown, 120
Mirapex, 84
Mirtazapine, 122–123
    for depression, 24
    for dissociative identity
        disorder, 26
Miss Emma, 200
Moban, 124
for conduct disorder, 18
for paranoia, 39
for schizophrenia, 49
Moban Concentrate, 124
Modafinil, 35, 123
Modecate, 132
Modecate Concentrate, 132
Moditen Enanthate, 132
Moditen HCl, 132
Moditen HCl-H.P., 132
Mogadon, 92, 173
Molindone, 123

for anxiety disorder, 14
for conduct disorder, 18
for paranoia, 39
for schizophrenia, 49
Monitan, 94
Monkey, 200
Monoamine oxidase inhibitors
    (MAOIs), 116–118
    for depression, 24
    for dissociative identity
        disorder, 26
    for panic disorder, 38
    for personality disorders,
        43
Mood, 225
Mood stabilizer, 254
Moon Gas, 194
Morph, 200
Morphine, 200
Morphitec, 200
M.O.S., 200
M.O.S.-SR, 200
Motion Aid, 85
Motion sickness, antihistamines
    for, 84–86
Movergan, 135
MS Contin, 200
MSIR, 200
MST Continus, 200
Mudrane GG, 90, 171
Multipax, 112
Murder 8, 185
Muscle spasms/strains
    benzodiazepines for, 91–93,
        172–174
    orphenadrine for, 128–129
    soma for, 213–215
Mushrooms, 203
Myolin, 128
Myotrol, 129
Myproic acid, 142
Mytussin AC, 179
Mytussin DAC, 179

N
Nadolol, 94
Naltrexone, 126, 166
Narcolepsy, 35

Novo-Tripramine, 82
Novotriptyn, 82
Novoxapam, 92, 173
Nozinan, 132
Nozinan Liquid, 132
Nozinan Oral Drops, 132
Nu-Alpraz, 92, 173
Nucochem, 179
Nucochem Expectorant, 179
Nucochem Pediatric Expectorant,
     179
Nucofed, 180
Nucofed Expectorant, 180
Nucofed Pediatric Expectorant,
     180
Nu-Loraz, 92, 173
Nu-Metop, 94
Nursing home abuse, 244,
     247–248
Nystagmus, 254
Nytol Maximum Strength, 85
Nytol with DPH, 85

O
OB, 216
Obesity, amphetamines for,
     80–81, 168–169
Obsession(s), 36, 254
Obsessive compulsive disorder
     (OCD), 36–37
   benzodiazepines for, 91–93,
     172–174
   buspirone for, 98
   lithium for, 114–115
   SSRIs for, 136–137
   tricyclic antidepressants for,
     82–83
O-Flex, 129
Olanzapine, 128
   for bipolar disorder, 16
   for conduct disorder, 18
   for paranoia, 40
   for schizophrenia, 49
   for Tourette's disorder, 55
Olfactory, 254
Omni-Tuss, 180
On-scene reports, 236
Open-ended questions, 4

Opium, 207–209
Oppositional defiant disorder
     (ODD), 37–38
Oral surgery, cocaine for, 176–178
Oramorph, 200
Oramorph-SR, 200
Orap, 84
Orflagen, 129
Orfro, 129
Oriented Times Four, 254
Orphenadrine, 41, 128–129
Orphenate, 129
Osteoporosis
   anabolic steroids for, 215–217
   definition of, 254
Overactivity in children
   clonidine for, 103–104
   guanfacine for, 110
Over-the-counter definition,
     254
Oxandrolone, 215
Oxazepam, 91, 172
Oxprenolol, 94
Oxy, 204
Oxycocet, 204
Oxycodone, 204
Oxycodone and acetaminophen,
     204
Oxycontin SR, 204
Oxy-Cotton, 204
Oxydess, 80, 168
Oxymetholone, 215
Oz, 194

P
Pacaps, 90, 171
Pain
   carbamazepine for, 99–100
   codeine for, 179–182
   marijuana for, 196–199
   morphine for, 200–202
   narcotic analgesics for,
     204–206
   opium for, 207–209
   trazodone for, 140–141
   tricyclic antidepressants
     for, 83
Pain Killers, 204

Psychosocial history, 223–224, 230–232
  definition of, 255
Psychotic, definition of, 255
Psychotropic medications, 60–80. *See also specific medications*
PTSD. *See* Post-traumatic stress disorder
Puberty, delayed, anabolic steroids for, 215–217
Pumpers, 216
Purple Passion, 203

**Q**

Quazepam, 91, 172
Quetiapine, 133–134
  for conduct disorder, 18
  for paranoia, 40
  for schizophrenia, 49

**R**

R2, 212
Razadyne, 102
  for Alzheimer's, 12
  for dementia, 23
R-Ball, 210
Red Birds, 171
Red Devils, 183
Redge, 197
Reds, 171
Rela, 212
Remeron, 122
  for depression, 24
  for dissociative identity disorder, 26
Remeron SolTab, 122
Repan, 90, 171
Reporting, 236–248
  of child abuse, 237–241
  of dependent adult abuse, 245–248
  of elder abuse, 241–244
Requip, 84
Restoril, 92, 173
ReVia, 126
Rhotrimine, 82
Rimantadine, 86
Risperdal, 134

Risperidone, 134
  for conduct disorder, 18
  for paranoia, 40
  for schizophrenia, 49
  for Tourette's disorder, 55
Ritalin, 121, 210
  for attention deficit disorders, 11
  for depression, 24
  for narcolepsy, 35
Ritalin LA, 121, 210
Ritalin SR, 121, 210
Rivastigmine, 102
Rivotril, 92, 173
RMS Uniserts, 200
Robafen AC Cough, 180
Robafen DAC, 180
Robitussin, 183
Robitussin A-C, 180
Robitussin-DAC, 180
Robo, 183
Robo Fry, 183
Roche, 212
Rock, 177
Rocket Fuel, 209
Rocks, 204
Rohypnol, 51, 212–213
Roids, 216
Rojo, 183
Rolatuss Expectorant, 180
Roll, 184
Rolling, 184
Roniacol, 127
Ronigen, 127
Roofies, 212
Roofinol, 212
Rope, 212
Ropinirole, 83
Round Ball, 210
Roxanol, 200
Roxanol SR, 200
Roxicet, 204
Roxicodone, 204
Roxilox, 204
Rush, 194
Rycotin, 127
Ryna-C Liquid, 180
Ryna-CX Liquid, 180

# NOTES

# NOTES

# NOTES

# NOTES

# NOTES

# NOTES

# NOTES

# NOTES

# NOTES

# NOTES

# NOTES